Essentials of Clinical Examination

Essentials of Clinical Examination:

A question and answer guide for students

Donald G. McLarty
Professor of Medicine
Muhimbili Medical Centre
Faculty of Medicine
Dar-es-Salaam
Tanzania

Baillière Tindall
London Philadelphia Toronto Sydney Tokyo

| Baillière Tindall | 24–28 Oval Road |
| W.B. Saunders | London NW1 7DX, UK |

The Curtis Center
Independence Square West
Philadelphia, PA 19106–3399, USA

55 Horner Avenue
Toronto, Ontario M8Z 4X6, Canada

Harcourt Brace Jovanovich Group (Australia) Pty Ltd
30–52 Smidmore Street
Marrickville
NSW 2204, Australia

Harcourt Brace Jovanovich Japan Inc
Ichibancho Central Building, 22–1 Ichibancho
Chiyoda-ku, Tokyo 102, Japan

© 1990 Baillière Tindall

Typeset by Colset Private Limited, Singapore

Printed and bound in Great Britain by Mackays of Chatham PLC, Chatham, Kent

British Library Cataloguing in Publication Data is available

ISBN 0-7020-1512-1

CONTENTS

To Dorothy, Pia and Ronald

PREFACE

'Where is the wisdom we have lost in knowledge?'
'Where is the knowledge we have lost in information?'

T.S. Eliot

This text was first produced for local use by students in the Faculty of Medicine, University of Dar-es-Salaam. The stimulus for preparing it arose from repeated encounters with undergraduates in clinical examinations, during which apparently many did not have the basic theoretical knowledge of clinical examination on which to base clinical skills, and interpret clinical findings.

The reasons for this lack of knowledge were related, in part, to a lack of basic textbooks, to overdependence on laboratory investigations, but, mainly, I believe, to a lack of appreciation of what they should and must know for competent clinical examination.

The problem of what should be known and how to set priorities when faced with an ever-increasing volume of medical information is a problem faced by medical students world-wide. Textbooks on clinical examination and medicine get progressively larger with each new edition, and undergraduates with limited clinical experience and, in many parts of the world, limited access to the guidance of teachers, find it difficult to see the wood for the trees.

This little book is one person's opinion of what represents an essential foundation of knowledge for acceptable clinical examination, and interpretation of clinical findings. It should be of relevance to undergraduates in both developing and developed countries, since the principles of physical examination are universal. The frequency of medical conditions does, of course, vary between developing and developed countries, and this has, at times, raised problems on what information should be included in the text and what left out. I hope, however, that a reasonable balance has been struck and that students everywhere will feel comfortable with the contents.

The book contains nothing new. It has been written, as Raymond y Cajal has said 'standing on other men's shoulders'. It is not intended to be a substitute for standard textbooks on methods of clinical examination, but should be seen as complementary and a means for students to test their knowledge, and quickly revise the essentials of clinical examination. It can also be used as a source of reference in the ward as the student begins to learn the skills of history taking and examination.

The idea for the catechismal presentation arose simply because knowledge is most commonly tested in response to questions, and a belief that this approach to learning is useful and valid. This approach may meet with the disapproval of many teachers who believe that it may discourage independent and logical thinking. Whatever one's view it remains that, for the successful completion of most tasks from driving a car to examination of the heart, certain facts must be known and rules followed. In addition, answering questions in the process of learning may enhance rather than discourage logical thinking. The questions, for example, on clinical findings in various clinical conditions require the student to think through the signs in a logical way as they proceed through the classic clinical steps of inspection, palpation, percussion and auscultation.

Many of the questions may seem excessively simple, but experience has shown that it is often the basic and simple facts that cause students to stumble. The same observation applies to postgraduate students, and they may find the book of value in revision of their basic knowledge of clinical examination. If many of the questions are considered too basic or irritating, they can be ignored, and the book read as a normal text.

In spite of the many advances of investigative medicine, clinical examination will continue to be of fundamental importance. This small book has been prepared in the hope that undergraduates will use it, as just one tool, in the improvement of their clinical skills.

Nothing has been mentioned in the text about the importance of correct attitudes as students begin and continue to relate
to patients. Suffice to say that if the golden rule, to treat others
as we ourselves would like to be treated, is remembered always,
few problems should arise in this area of clinical examination.

D.G. McLarty

ACKNOWLEDGEMENTS

Tribute has already been expressed in the Preface to the authors of papers and textbooks on clinical examination and Internal Medicine from which the contents of this book have been drawn. Books referred to included *Hutchison's Clinical Methods* by Swash and Mason, *Clinical Examination* by MacLeod, *A Primer of Medicine* by Pappworth, Davidson's *Principles and Practice of Medicine, Clinical Medicine* edited by Kumar and Clark, and *Aids to the Examination of the Peripheral Nervous System*, HMSO. The questions which may be asked of a patient who may have AIDS were described in an article by Diana Antoniskis, Fred R. Sattler and John M. Leedom, in *Postgraduate Medicine*.

Mrs Frances White, Ms Esther I. Kawogo, Ms Piazis Kopwe and Dr Andrew Swai provided invaluable help in the typing and preparation of the manuscript. Dr Charles Tomson read the first draft and made many useful suggestions. Special thanks are also due to many others who provided valuable advice. Dr Paul McGill assisted with the section on examination of the joints and Dr Basil Schofield with the section dealing with examination of patients with sexually transmitted diseases. Thanks are also due to Professor K.G.M.M. Alberti for his support and encouragement. The idea for the book came from the Shorter Catechism of the Free Church of Scotland.

All royalties from this book will go towards the provision of text-books for medical students in sub-Saharan Africa.

References

1. Swash M. ed. *Hutchison's Clinical Methods*. 19th ed. London: Baillière Tindall, 1989.

2. MacLeod, J. ed. *Clinical Examination*. 5th ed. Edinburgh: Churchill Livingstone, 1979.

3. Pappworth, M.H. *A Primer of Medicine*. 5th ed. London: Butterworths, 1984.

4. MacLeod, J. ed. *Davidson's Principles & Practice of Medicine*. 14th ed. Edinburgh: Churchill Livingstone, 1984.

5. Kumar, P.J., Clark, M.L. eds. *Clinical Medicine*. 2nd ed. London: Baillière Tindall, 1990.

6. Medical Research Council. *Aids to the Examination of the Peripheral Nervous System*. Memorandum No. 45. London: HMSO, 1975.

7. Antoniskis, D., Sattler, F.R., Leedom, J.M. Importance of assessing risk behaviour for AIDS. Why and how to obtain a relevant history. *Postgraduate Medicine* (1988) **83**, 138–150.

1
THE CARDIOVASCULAR SYSTEM

SYMPTOMATIC ENQUIRY IN PATIENTS WITH CARDIOVASCULAR DISEASE

Q1.1 What are the cardinal symptoms of heart disease?

A:
- Breathlessness.
- Chest pain.
- Oedema.
- Palpitations.

Q1.2 What are other important symptoms of heart disease?

A:
- Fatigue.[1]
- Syncope.[2]

1. Fatigue or tiredness is due, at least in part, to a low cardiac output with resulting poor cerebral and peripheral perfusion. Drugs, e.g. beta-blockers, may also contribute.
2. See Q1.12.

Q1.3 What are the symptoms of peripheral vascular disease?

A:
- Pain in the calves on exercise (intermittent claudication).[1]
- Coldness of the feet.
- Rest pain in the muscles of the legs or feet at rest.
- Leg ulcers and gangrene.

1. Some patients may complain of pain in the buttocks on walking due to stenosis at the bifurcation of the aorta.

BREATHLESSNESS

Q1.4 What features should be noted about breathlessness?

A: • If it occurs on exertion or at rest.
   • If patient is wakened at night by breathlessness (paroxysmal nocturnal dyspnoea).
   • If it occurs when lying flat (orthopnoea).
   • Duration.
   • Severity, e.g. how far can patient walk? How many stairs can be climbed before onset of breathlessness?
   • Precipitating factors.

Q1.5 The New York Heart Association's functional classification provides information of the extent to which a patient is limited by symptoms of heart disease.[1] **Describe the classification.**

A: Class 1 – asymptomatic (no functional limitation).
   Class 2 – symptomatic on extra exertion.
   Class 3 – symptomatic on mild exertion.
   Class 4 – symptomatic at rest or on minimal exertion (severe functional limitation).

   1. The degree of limitation is generally related to disease severity and prognosis.

Q1.6 How may the severity of orthopnoea be assessed?

A: By the number of pillows used.

CHEST PAIN

Q1.7 What features should be noted about chest pain?

A: • Site.
   • Duration.
   • Character.[1]
   • Relieving factors.
   • Whether experienced on exertion or at rest.[2]

- Radiation.
- Accompanying sensations.[3]
- Precipitating factors.[4]

1. Sharp, crushing or tight.
2. Decubitus angina, for example, occurs when the patient lies down, and nocturnal angina wakens the patient from sleep. Variant (Prinzmetal's) angina also commonly occurs at rest as does unstable angina.
3. Cold sweats, nausea and vomiting.
4. Emotion, heavy meal, cold, etc.

Q1.8 What causes of chest pain should be differentiated from the pain of angina of effort?

A:
- Pleurisy.[1]
- Pericarditis.[1]
- Precordial catch.[2]
- Chronic pulmonary embolism; pulmonary infarction.
- Pulmonary hypertension.
- Oesophageal spasm or reflux.
- Costochondritis.
- Dissecting aneurysm.
- Anxiety and hypochondria.
- Asthma.

1. Pain is aggravated by movement, respiration and coughing. The pain of pleurisy is felt laterally and the pain of pericarditis is usually felt in the centre of the chest.
2. Also known as effort (Da Costa's) syndrome. The patient complains of left-sided submammary stabbing pain, often associated with anxiety. Mitral valve prolapse can cause a similar kind of pain.

Q1.9 What causes of chest pain should be differentiated from the pain of acute myocardial infarction?

A:
- Massive pulmonary embolism.
- Dissecting aneurysm.
- Oesophageal spasm.
- Pneumothorax.

- Perforated or bleeding peptic ulcer.
- Pancreatitis.

PALPITATIONS

Q1.10 Palpitations may be experienced when the patient is anxious, lying on the left side or after exercise. **What are the most common arrhythmias associated with palpitations?**

A: • Premature ectopic beats.
• Paroxysmal tachycardias.

Q1.11 How may palpitations be graded?

A: Grade 0 – asymptomatic.
Grade 1 – non-sustained palpitations.
Grade 2 – sustained palpitations.
Grade 3 – palpitations and other symptoms (e.g. dyspnoea, chest pain, dizziness).
Grade 4 – syncope.

SYNCOPE

Q1.12 Most syncopal attacks (faints) are vasovagal in nature, and are not due to cardiac disease. **What are the main causes of cardiovascular syncope?**[1]

A: • Heart block (Adams – Stokes attacks).
• Ventricular tachycardia.
• Rapid supraventricular tachycardia.
• Aortic stenosis.
• Hypertrophic obstructive cardiomyopathy.

1. Cardiovascular syncope should be suspected if syncope occurs during exercise or in the absence of a clear precipitating cause.

Q1.13 Are symptoms always present in patients with severe cardiac disease?

A: No – patients, e.g. with severe mitral stenosis or hypertension may be symptomless. Hence the need for careful routine examination.

PAST MEDICAL HISTORY, SOCIAL AND FAMILY HISTORY

Q1.14 In the past medical history, and social and family history, what points should be noted?

A:
- History of acute rheumatic fever, joint pains, recurrent sore throats, hypertension or blood diseases.
- Current drug treatment.
- Smoking.
- Alcohol intake.
- Occupation and socioeconomic status.[1]

1. How has illness affected patient's ability to work, and what will its impact be on patient's future?

GENERAL EXAMINATION

Q1.15 What general features should be noted in a patient with heart disease?

A:
- Anaemia.[1]
- Cachexia.
- Obesity.[2]
- Cyanosis – central and peripheral.[3]
- Hepatomegaly.[4]
- Finger clubbing.[5]
- Evidence of thyroid disease.

1. May exacerbate existing heart failure.
2. Obesity may be associated with hypertension, heart disease, breathlessness, stroke and hyperlipidaemia.
3. Central cyanosis indicates right-to-left shunting of the blood in the heart and great vessels, or passage of blood through the lungs without adequate oxygenation, e.g. in emphysema. Peripheral cyanosis with cold extremities suggests a low cardiac output.
4. May be a sign of right heart failure.
5. May be found in cyanotic congenital heart disease and infective endocarditis. Clubbing occuring in cor pulmonale is usually associated with the underlying lung disease, e.g. fibrosing alveolitis.

Q1.16 What general features may be found in a patient with infective endocarditis?

A:
- Fever.
- Anaemia.
- Cachexia.
- Finger clubbing.
- Petechial or mucosal haemorrhages.[1]
- Splinter haemorrhages in the nail beds.[2]
- Osler's nodes.[3]
- Arthritis of major joints.
- Splenomegaly.[4]
- Haematuria.
- New heart murmur(s) or change in murmur(s)

1. Due to vasculitis.
2. Manifestation of microvascular embolic phenomena.
3. Painful erythematous lumps in the pulps of fingers and toes, palms of the hand and soles of the feet – another embolic manifestation in infective endocarditis which is rarely seen.
4. Slight splenomegaly is common.

PALPATION OF THE PULSE

Q1.17 In clinical practice the radial pulse is normally palpated, but abnormal features of the pulse may be best appreciated by palpation of the carotid artery. **When palpating the radial pulse what four features should always be noted?**

A: Rate, rhythm, volume and character.

Pulse Rate

Q1.18 What clinical conditions are most commonly associated with a tachycardia (pulse rate over 100 beats per minute)?

A:
- Emotion.
- Exercise.
- Pregnancy.
- Fever.

- Anaemia.
- Heart failure.
- Arrhythmias.
- Thyrotoxicosis.

Q1.19 What are the most important intracardiac causes of bradycardia? (Pulse rate less than 60 beats per minute)

A: • Sinus node disease (sick sinus syndrome).
  • Atrioventricular (AV) block.

Q1.20 Describe other causes of or clinical conditions associated with bradycardia

A: • Old age and in fit athletic persons.
  • Drug therapy.[1]
  • Hypothermia.
  • Hypothyroidism.
  • Cholestatic jaundice.
  • Raised intracranial pressure.

  1. Beta-blockers, digoxin and other antiarrhythmic drugs.

Rhythm of pulse

Q1.21 What is meant by the rhythm of the pulse?

A: Whether it is regular or irregular.

Q1.22 In which normal circumstance may the pulse appear to be irregular?

A: In sinus arrhythmia.

Q1.23 What is sinus arrhythmia?

A: A noticeable increase in pulse rate during inspiration, which is physiological and most commonly observed in children.

Q1.24 What are the two most common causes of an irregular rhythm?

A: 1. Atrial fibrillation.
  2. Ventricular ectopic beats (extrasystoles).

Q1.25 How, clinically, can you distinguish between atrial fibrillation and ventricular extrasystoles?

A: When frequent extrasystoles are the cause of the irregular rhythm the underlying rhythm can usually be appreciated as being regular, whereas in atrial fibrillation the rhythm is completely irregular and the beats are unequal in volume. In atrial fibrillation there will also be a pulse deficit, i.e. the heart rate counted at the apex will be greater than the rate counted at the wrist.[1]

1. A pulse deficit results from the varying length of diastole in atrial fibrillation. Short diastole results in inadequate filling of ventricles and low stroke volume so that the pulse wave is not recorded at the wrist. A pulse deficit is, of course, not unique to atrial fibrillation and may occur with any rapid arrhythmia. For exact determination of the cause of an irregular rhythm an electrocardiogram is necessary.

Q1.26 What are the main causes of atrial fibrillation?

A: • Rheumatic heart disease.
    • Ischaemic heart disease.
    • Alcohol.
    • Thyrotoxicosis.

Pulse Volume or Pulse Pressure

Q1.27 What is meant by the pulse volume?

A: The pulse volume refers to the strength of the pulse wave.

Q1.28 What factors determine pulse volume?

A: • The anatomy of the aortic valve (narrowed or dilated).
    • Cardiac output.
    • The state of the vessel walls.

Q1.29 What adjectives are used to describe the pulse volume?

A: Large, normal or small, or high, normal or low.

Q1.30 Name some clinical conditions which may be associated with a small volume pulse

A: • State of shock due to blood loss, etc.
    • Congestive cardiac failure.
    • Aortic stenosis.
    • Constrictive pericarditis.
    • Severe mitral stenosis.

Q1.31 What common clinical conditions may be associated with a large volume pulse?

A: • Certain febrile states.
    • Anaemia.
    • Thyrotoxicosis.
    • Aortic regurgitation.

Character of Pulse Wave

Q1.32 What is meant by the character of the pulse?

A: By character of the pulse we mean whether it is normal, collapsing, i.e. quick rising/quick falling, or a plateau pulse, i.e. slow rising/slow falling. A plateau pulse is sometimes referred to as an anacrotic pulse.

Q1.33 What is meant by a collapsing pulse, and with what conditions can it be associated?

A: A collapsing pulse is a large volume, quick rising quick falling pulse which occurs in states in which there is increased cardiac output, e.g. pregnancy, fever, patent ductus arteriosus. It is, however, particularly associated with aortic regurgitation.

Q1.34 How can a collapsing pulse best be demonstrated?

A: By placing the palm of the examiner's hand over the anterior aspect of the patient's wrist and then elevating the patient's arm. The pulse volume increases on elevation of the arm.

Q1.35 With which heart valve lesion is an anacrotic or plateau pulse associated?

A: Aortic stenosis.

Other Kinds of Pulse

Q1.36 What is pulsus bigeminus (coupled beat)?

A: A ventricular extrasystole occurring after every normal heart beat. It is often due to digoxin toxicity.

Q1.37 What is pulsus alternans?

A: Pulsus alternans refers to alternating high and low volume beats. It is best appreciated by using a sphygmomanometer, and is an important sign of left ventricular failure.

Q1.38 What is pulsus paradoxus?

A: Pulsus parodoxus is misleadingly named.[1] It is an exaggeration of the normal decrease in arterial pressure[2] and pulse volume which accompanies inspiration. It may be detected by palpation of the radial pulse, but is best appreciated by the use of a sphygmomanometer. It is associated with pericardial effusion and constrictive pericarditis. It also occurs in severe asthma.

1. The 'paradox' relates to the clinical finding of heart sounds heard on auscultation over the precordium when no pulse is palpable at the wrist.
2. Not more than 5 mmHg.

Q1.39 What is pulsus bisferiens?

A: Pulsus bisferiens is a double beat, best felt in the internal carotid artery in combined aortic stenosis and regurgitation. It may also be felt in hypertrophic obstructive cardiomyopathy.

BLOOD PRESSURE

Q1.40 Systolic pressure is the pressure at which the first Korotkov sound is heard when auscultating over the brachial artery. **How is diastolic pressure recorded?**

A: Diastolic pressure may be recorded either when the Korotkov sounds suddenly become muffled (phase 4) or when they disappear (phase 5).

Q1.41 In clinical practice usually only phase 5 is recorded. What is the value of also recording phase 4?

A: Sometimes sounds do not disappear completely, and the recording of phase 5 is difficult. It is therefore of value to practise recording both phase 4 and phase 5.

Q1.42 With what degree of accuracy should blood pressure be measured?

A: To the nearest 2 mmHg.

Q1.43 Will using a standard arm cuff size (12 cm) in an obese patient lead to under- or overestimation of the blood pressure?

A: Overestimation.

ARTERIES

Q1.44 Apart from palpation of the radial artery, which other arterial pulses should be examined on routine clinical examination?

A: The internal carotid arteries, and the major arteries of the lower limb, especially the femoral, posterior tibial and dorsalis pedis arteries.

Q1.45 What is the value of auscultation over arteries?

A: In peripheral vascular disease bruits may be audible over areas of stenosis in large arteries. Bruits may also be heard in renal artery stenosis. In aortic regurgitation 'pistol shot' sounds are heard on auscultation over the femoral arteries.

VEINS

Q1.46 What two clinical conditions may be associated with non-pulsatile venous distension in (1) the neck and upper anterior part of chest, and (2) the abdomen?

A: 1. Superior mediastinal obstruction.
2. Hepatic cirrhosis with portal hypertension.

VENOUS PRESSURE

Q1.47 Why is assessment of venous pressure important?

A: An elevated venous pressure is one of the most important signs of heart failure.

Q1.48 What other conditions are associated with elevation of the jugular venous pressure?

A: • Constrictive pericarditis.
• Cardiac tamponade.
• Overtransfusion of fluids.
• Superior vena caval obstruction.[1]

1. In this condition venous pulsation will be absent.

Q1.49 How do you determine evidence of raised venous pressure?

A: By inspection of the neck veins.

Q1.50 How do you distinguish between venous and arterial pulsations?

A: Venous pulsations have a rippling or undulating appearance, and a double peak[1] can often be seen. Unlike arterial pulses they are usually not palpable.

1. The double peak is due to the 'a' wave (atrial systole) and the 'v' wave is just prior to the opening of the tricuspid valve. The venous pulse has three positive waves but the 'c' wave is rarely visible.

Q1.51 Which vein is used to determine venous pressure?

A: The internal jugular vein.

Q1.52 Where should the internal jugular vein be looked for?

A: On a line joining the sternoclavicular joint to the angle of the jaw.

Q1.53 Is it not easier to use the external jugular vein?

A: Yes, but the external jugular vein is easily distended in some normal individuals by slight neck movements. It should only be used if the normal venous pulsations are visible, indicating absence of obstruction to flow.

Q1.54 Is it always possible to visualize the internal jugular vein in patients with congestive cardiac failure?

A: Sometimes it can be difficult and one may have to rely on the external jugular vein.[1]

1. If the jugular venous pressure is markedly elevated, the top of the column of blood where pulsation is most striking may be in the cranium. If you suspect this to be the the case sit the patient upright.

Q1.55 How should the patient be positioned for examination of jugular venous pressure (JVP)?

A: At an angle of approximately 45°.

Q1.56 How is venous pressure recorded?

A: By recording the vertical height of the venous column above the sternal angle.

Q1.57 Where is the sternal angle?

A: The junction of the manubrium sternum with the sternal body at the junction of the second costal cartilage.

Q1.58 If you suspect that your patient is in congestive cardiac failure, but are uncertain from direct inspection of neck veins, what other procedure can you perform to enable you to assess increased venous pressure?

A: Look for evidence of hepatojugular reflux by pressing gently over the abdomen.[1]

1. Pressure over the abdomen causes an increase in central and jugular venous pressure. The normal heart will quickly compensate by an increase in cardiac output. The failing heart, however, cannot compensate quickly and jugular venous pressure remains elevated.

Abnormal Venous Pulse Waveforms in Neck Veins

Q1.59 What are cannon waves?

A: Large 'a' waves which are most commonly associated with complete heart block when the atrium contracts against a closed tricuspid valve. They may also be seen in ventricular tachycardia and in patients with right ventricular hypertrophy due, for example, to pulmonary hypertension. In right ventricular hypertrophy there is increased resistance to filling.

Q1.60 What may be seen in tricuspid incompetence?

A: Giant systolic or 'v' waves.

Q1.61 What is Kussmaul's sign?

A: Elevation of the jugular venous pressure with inspiration.

Q1.62 What clinical condition is associated with Kussmaul's sign?

A: Pericardial effusion or constrictive pericarditis, which cause obstruction to venous filling of the heart.

Q1.63 What is Freidreich's sign?

A: The rapid fall and rise of the jugular venous pulse which may occur in constrictive pericarditis and tricuspid regurgitation.

OEDEMA

Q1.64 Where should you look for 'pitting' oedema in patients in congestive cardiac failure?

A: In the lumbosacral area (especially if patient is recumbent) and in the legs and feet.

EXAMINATION OF THE HEART

Q1.65 How should you proceed to examine the heart?

A: By inspection, palpation and auscultation.

Q1.66 What should you look for on inspection?

A: • Deformities of the chest which might affect the heart's function and position.[1]
   • The position of the cardiac (apical) impulse, whether localized or diffuse.
   • The presence of other pulsations in the chest, in the epigastrium and right hypochondrium.

   1. Kyphoscoliosis, for example, may both affect position of the apex beat and cause an ejection systolic murmur.

PALPATION

Q1.67 What signs should be looked for by palpation?

A: • Position and character of the apex beat.
   • Presence of thrills.
   • Parasternal heave.

Position of the Apex Beat

Q1.68 How is the apex beat defined?

A: That point on the chest wall furthest outwards and downwards where the cardiac impulse can be distinctly felt.

Q1.69 How is the apex beat measured?

A: From the mid-line.

Q1.70 Where does it normally lie?

A: In the fifth intercostal space 9 cm or less from the midline in upright adults, just within the mid-clavicular line.

Q1.71 How may the apex be shifted in position?

A:
- By skeletal abnormalities, e.g. kyphoscoliosis.
- By changes of posture.
- By increase in the size of the heart.
- By changes in the lungs.
- Dextrocardia.

Q1.72 What lung conditions may change the position of the apex?

A:
- Pleural effusion or pneumothorax in the right lung may displace the apex laterally, i.e. away from the side of the lesion.
- Collapse (atelectasis) and fibrosis in the right lung may displace the apex medially, i.e. towards the side of the lesion.

Character of Apex

Q1.73 What is meant by the character of the apex beat?

A:
- Whether localized or diffuse.
- Whether heaving or thrusting, or tapping.
- Whether associated with a thrill.

Q1.74 With what cardiac condition is a heaving/thrusting apex beat associated?

A: Left ventricular hypertrophy.[1]

1. A heaving or sustained pulsation is usually associated with systemic hypertension and aortic stenosis ('pressure overload'), whilst a thrusting or non-sustained pulsation is commonly due to mitral and aortic regurgitation ('volume overload'). In practice it is often difficult to distinguish between these two types of pulsation.

Q1.75 What does a tapping apex signify?

A: Abnormal closure of mitral valve in mitral stenosis, i.e. a palpable first heart sound.

Q1.76 What conditions may be associated with a double apex beat, i.e. two pulsations with each heart beat?

A: • Hypertrophic cardiomyopathy.
   • Ventricular aneurysm.

Q1.77 If the apex beat is not palpable what could be the cause?

A: • Obesity.
   • Pericardial effusion.
   • Emphysema.

Thrills

Q1.78 What is a thrill?

A: A thrill is a palpable murmur.

Q1.79 Is a thrill palpated at the apex likely to be systolic or diastolic?

A: Diastolic, associated with mitral stenosis.

Q1.80 Is a thrill palpated at the base of the heart likely to be systolic or diastolic?

A: Systolic, associated with pulmonary stenosis or aortic stenosis.

Q1.81 In which other sites can the thrill of aortic stenosis be palpated?

A: Carotid arteries and suprasternal notch.

Left Parasternal Heave

Q1.82 What is the significance of a left parasternal heave?

A: It often indicates (1) right ventricular hypertrophy, as in mitral stenosis, (2) right ventricular dilatation as in atrial septal defect, or (3) hypertrophy or enlargement of the left atrium. The most common cause of a parasternal heave in practice is mitral regurgitation, which leads to systolic expansion of the left atrium.

Percussion

Q1.83 Is percussion of the heart of value in clinical examination?

A: Percussion of the heart to determine its size is inaccurate. Cardiac size is best assessed by palpation of the position of the apex beat.

AUSCULTATION

Q1.84 When auscultating the heart what are you listening for?

A: • The heart sounds.
   • Murmurs.
   • Pericardial friction.

Q1.85 What are the four standard areas for auscultation?

A: 1. Aortic area – second right intercostal space, just to the right of the sternum.
   2. Pulmonary area – second left intercostal space, just to the left of the sternum.
   3. Tricuspid area – left border of the sternum at its lower end, in the fourth intercostal space.
   4. Mitral area – apex of heart.

Q1.86 Should auscultation be limited to these areas?

A: No, murmurs may often be heard best at the left sternal border (aortic regurgitation), the lower right parasternal area (tricuspid regurgitation and stenosis), just medial to the apex (mitral stenosis), the axilla (mitral regurgitation) and the carotids (aortic stenosis).

Q1.87 How may the heart sounds be altered?

A: They may be loud or soft, or split.

Heart Sounds

The first heart sound

Q1.88 What is the origin of the first heart sound?

A: Abrupt closure of the mitral and tricuspid valves.[1]

    1. The tricuspid component is minor.

Q1.89 What conditions are associated with a loud first heart sound?

A: Mitral stenosis and a hyperdynamic circulation due, for example, to anaemia or thyrotoxicosis.

Q1.90 What conditions are associated with a soft first heart sound?

A:
- Acute rheumatic fever.
- Mitral regurgitation.
- Calcific mitral stenosis.
- After myocardial infarction.
- Heart failure.
- Cardiogenic shock.
- Pericardial effusion.
- Obesity.
- Emphysema.

Q1.91 What conditions may be associated with variation in intensity of the first heart sound?

A: Ventricular tachycardia[1] and complete heart block when atrial and ventricular systole is asynchronous.[1]

    1. The first heart sound is soft if the P–R interval is long, and loud when the P–R interval is short.

Q1.92 What does splitting of the heart sounds mean?

A: That contraction of the two ventricles is not quite synchronous. Splitting of the heart sounds is usually a normal finding.

Q1.93 Where is splitting of the first sound best heard?

A: In the tricuspid area.

The Second Heart Sound

Q1.94 What is the origin of the second heart sound?

A: Aortic and pulmonary valve closure.

Q1.95 In what conditions is the second heart sound decreased?

A: • Aortic stenosis.
   • Heart failure.
   • Pulmonary stenosis.

Q1.96 In what conditions is the second heart sound accentuated?

A: • In systemic hypertension at the aortic area.
   • In pulmonary hypertension over the pulmonary area.

Q1.97 Does inspiration increase or decrease splitting of the second heart sound?

A: Increase – closure of the pulmonary valve is delayed in inspiration.

Q1.98 Where is the splitting of the second heart sound heard best?

A: In the pulmonary area.

Q1.99 In what conditions does wide splitting of the second sound occur?

A: • Bundle-branch block.
   • Pulmonary stenosis.

Q1.100 What is meant by a 'fixed split'?

A: No change in splitting on respiration.

Q1.101 Name two conditions in which fixed splitting occurs

A: 1. Right bundle-branch block.
2. Atrial septal defect.

Q1.102 What is meant by reversed or paradoxical splitting of heart sounds?

A: Splitting of the heart sounds in which the pulmonary component comes before the aortic component, and in which splitting decreases on inspiration.

Q1.103 In what conditions may a reversed split be observed?

A: • Left bundle-branch block.
• Left ventricular failure.
• Severe aortic stenosis.
• Patent ductus arteriosus.

The Third Heart Sound
Q1.104 What causes the third heart sound?

A: Rapid ventricular filling when the tricuspid and mitral valves open. It therefore occurs early in diastole just after the second sound.

Q1.105 Is an audible third heart sound normal or abnormal?

A: It is often present normally in children, young adults and in pregnancy but may also have pathological significance.

Q1.106 In what pathological conditions might you hear a third heart sound?

A: In conditions in which there is rapid ventricular filling, e.g. heart failure, mitral regurgitation and ventricular septal defect.

The Fourth Heart Sound
Q1.107 What is the fourth heart sound?

A: The fourth heart sound is due to ventricular filling after atrial contraction. It therefore occurs just before the first heart sound. It should be distinguished from splitting of the first heart sound. It occurs when the left ventricle is under strain, or as a result of hypertension or following myocardial infarction. Remember that it will be absent in the presence of atrial fibrillation.

Gallop Rhythm
Q1.108 What is a gallop or triple rhythm?

A: A rapid heart rate with a third or fourth heart sound, or both.

Q1.109 With what condition is a gallop rhythm associated?

A: Cardiac failure.

Q1.110 Is it always easy to distinguish between a third and fourth heart sound?

A: No, especially when there is a tachycardia. Clinically, it is not important if one cannot. What is more important is to be able to distinguish between the first heart sound and an opening snap.

Opening Snap
Q1.111 What is an opening snap?

A: An opening snap is a sound heard just after the first heart sound in mitral stenosis. It is caused by opening of the diseased mitral valve.

Ejection click
Q1.112 What is an ejection click?

A: A sharp, high-pitched sound in early systole which is sometimes heard in aortic stenosis, pulmonary stenosis and hypertension.

Pericardial 'knock'?

Q1.113 What is a pericardial 'knock'?

A: A loud diastolic sound heard during diastole in constrictive pericarditis. It is related to the abrupt halt to diastolic filling which occurs in this condition.

Murmurs

Q1.114 What are murmurs and what causes them?

A: Murmurs are sounds additional to the heart sounds. They usually result from turbulent blood flow either:

- Where blood flow is increased through a normal valve.
- Where blood is forced through a narrowed valve orifice.
- Where blood regurgitates through an incompetent or 'leaky' valve.
- Where blood is passing through an abnormal communication between the chambers of the heart, or great arteries, e.g. ventricular septal defect and patent ductus arteriosus.

Q1.115 Are murmurs therefore always of pathological significance?

A: No. Sometimes systolic murmurs may be heard in the absence of any abnormality of the heart. They are termed 'innocent', 'functional' or 'benign'.

Q1.116 When are 'innocent' murmurs most commonly heard?

A: In hyperdynamic states such as pregnancy or anaemia.

Q1.117 What points should be noted when listening to a murmur?

A: • Timing, i.e. systolic or diastolic. Systolic murmurs occur between the first and second heart sounds and diastolic murmurs between the second and first sounds. The first heart sound can be identified by palpating the apex beat or the carotid arteries.

- Position, i.e. where murmur is heard loudest.
- Conduction, i.e. the directions in which the murmur can be followed and heard clearly.
- Intensity or loudness*. This can be graded 1 to 6 as follows:
  1 just audible;
  2 quiet;
  3 moderately loud;
  4 loud with palpable thrill;
  5 very loud with pronounced thrill;
  6 audible without aid of stethoscope.
- Character or quality – various terms are used to describe the character of murmurs such as high-pitched, low-pitched, rumbling, rough or blowing.
- Change of murmur with posture and during respiration – the more changeable a murmur, the less likely it is to be significant.

* Note that the loudness of a murmur does not always correlate with severity of the valve lesion. In aortic stenosis and mitral stenosis, for example, the duration of the murmur is a more reliable guide to severity.

Q1.118 What is the most common error encountered with regard to the timing of murmurs?

A: Confusing systole and diastole.[1]

1. Murmurs are best timed in relation to the first and second heart sounds.

Systolic Murmurs
Q1.119 How are systolic murmurs classified?

A: Into (1) mid-systolic or 'ejection' murmurs and (2) pansystolic murmurs.

(i) Mid-systolic murmurs
Q1.120 Describe the cardiac lesions which are associated with a mid-systolic murmur[1]

A: • 'Innocent' or functional murmurs.
- Aortic stenosis – an often loud, low-pitched mid-systolic murmur best heard in the aortic area and which radiates into the neck and to the apex.

- Aortic sclerosis – a mid-systolic murmur similar to that of aortic stenosis.
- Pulmonary stenosis – a mid-systolic murmur best heard over the pulmonary area and left sternal edge.
- Mitral valve prolapse – a mid- to late systolic murmur best heard at the left sternal edge.
- Atrial septal defect – a mid-systolic murmur best heard at the left sternal edge.

1. Some mid-systolic or ejection murmurs are long and appear to continue up to second sound, e.g. severe aortic stenosis.

(ii) Pansystolic murmurs

Q1.121 Describe the cardiac lesions associated with a pansystolic murmur

A: • Mitral regurgitation – a pansystolic murmur best heard at the apex which radiates to the axilla and sometimes to the back.
- Ventricular septal defect – a pansystolic murmur best heard at the lower left sternal edge.
- Tricuspid regurgitation – a pansystolic murmur best heard at the lower right sternal edge, associated with hepatic pulsation and giant jugular 'v' waves.

Diastolic Murmurs:

(i) Early diastolic murmurs

Q1.122 Describe the valvular lesions associated with an early diastolic murmur

A: • Aortic regurgitation – an early diastolic murmur best heard at the left sternal edge with the diaphragm of the stethoscope, and with the patient sitting up, leaning forwards and holding the breath in expiration. It is often faint, blowing in quality and high pitched.
- Pulmonary regurgitation – an early diastolic murmur best heard in the pulmonary area. When associated with pulmonary hypertension due to mitral stenosis it is called a Graham Steell murmur.

(ii) Mid-diastolic murmurs

Q1.123 Describe the conditions associated with a mid-diastolic murmur

A: • Mitral stenosis – a low-pitched, rumbling, mid-diastolic murmur with presystolic accentuation if patient is in sinus rhythm. The murmur is best heard at or just medial to the apex with the bell of the stethoscope, and with the patient lying on the left side. An opening snap is usually hard just prior to or at the onset of the murmur.

• Austin Flint murmur – a diastolic murmur heard at the apex in patients with aortic regurgitation.[1]

• Carey Coombs murmur – a short diastolic murmur heard in acute rheumatic fever when there is involvement of the mitral valve.

1. In aortic regurgitation the regurgitation of blood into the left ventricle may partially obstruct the mitral valve.

Continuous Murmurs (Murmurs which Extend from Early Systole to Diastole)

Q1.124 What condition is most commonly associated with a continuous murmur?

A: Patent ductus arteriosus.

Q1.125 Where is the murmur best heard?

A: At the pulmonary area or below the left clavicle.

Pericardial Friction Rub

Q1.126 Describe the main features of a pericardial rub?

A: It is a superficial, creaky sound. It is usually heard in both systole and diastole and may vary with respiration and posture. It will not disappear on holding the breath whereas a pleuropericardial rub may.

OTHER SIGNS OF CARDIAC DISEASE

Q1.127 What other organs should be examined in a patient with cardiac disease?

A: • The lungs for the presence of crepitations or crackles.
   • The abdomen for evidence of hepatomegaly.
   • The fundi for evidence of hypertensive changes.

HEART FAILURE

Q1.128 How is cardiac failure classified clinically?[1]

A: • Right heart failure.
   • Left heart failure.
   • Congestive (biventricular) heart failure.

   1. Whilst this classification is useful in clinical practice, it is rather rare for the right or left heart to fail in isolation.

Q1.129 What are the common causes of right heart failure?

A: • Chronic lung disease (cor pulmonale).
   • Pulmonary embolism.
   • Pulmonary hypertension.[1]
   • Rheumatic heart disease involving the tricuspid valves.
   • Pulmonary stenosis.
   • Atrial and ventricular septal defects with left-to- right shunting of blood.

   1. Due, for example, to mitral stenosis.

Q1.130 What are the usual physical signs of right heart failure?

A: • Elevated jugular venous pressure.
   • Tachycardia.
   • Hepatomegaly.[1]
   • Ascites.
   • Ankle oedema.

- Gallop rhythm.[2]
- Pansystolic murmur.[3]

1. Tender and smooth.
2. A right ventricular third or fourth heart sound is commonly heard.
3. Dilatation of right ventricle may result in functional tricuspid valve regurgitation.

Q1.131 Name the common causes of left heart failure

A: • Ischaemic heart disease.
- Systemic hypertension.
- Cardiomyopathies.
- Disease of the mitral and aortic valves.
- Persistent patent ductus arteriosus.

Q1.132 What are the main physical signs of left heart failure?

A: • Cardiac enlargement.[1]
- Third or fourth heart sound audible.
- Crackles at lung bases or throughout lungs in severe left ventricular failure.

1. Not always obvious clinically.

Q1.133 What signs are associated with congestive (biventricular) cardiac failure?[1]

A: A combination of the signs associated with both right and left heart failure.

1. Congestive cardiac failure most commonly refers to the development of right heart failure secondary to previous left heart failure.

Q1.134 What conditions are associated with high output heart failure?

A: • Thyrotoxicosis.
- Beriberi.
- Systemic arteriovenous fistula.

- Gram-negative septicaemia.
- Paget's disease.

Q1.135 What conditions should be looked for in a patient with rheumatic heart disease who develops heart failure or whose existing heart failure becomes worse?

A: • Anaemia.
  • Arrhythmias.
  • Infective endocarditis.
  • Thyrotoxicosis.
  • Pregnancy.

RHEUMATIC FEVER

Q1.136 What are the revised Duckett- Jones criteria for the diagnosis of rheumatic fever?

A: 1. Major criteria:
  • Carditis.
  • Polyarthritis.
  • Chorea.
  • Erythema marginatum.
  • Subcutaneous nodules.
  2. Minor criteria:
  • Fever.
  • Arthralgia.
  • Previous rheumatic fever.
  • Raised ESR.
  • Leukocytosis.
  • Prolonged P–R interval on ECG.

Q1.137 What criteria are required for the diagnosis of rheumatic fever?[1]

A: • Two or more major criteria.
  • One major plus two or more minor criteria.

  1. Both sets of criteria should be accompanied by evidence of recent streptococcal infection, e.g. culture of group A streptococcus from throat swab, ASO titre >250

units or history of recent scarlet fever. In many developing countries the classic picture of acute rheumatic fever is seldom seen. The diagnosis of rheumatic fever should therefore be considered in children whose only complaint is joint pain or swelling.

Q1.138 What are the clinical manifestations of carditis?

A: • New or changing heart murmurs.
• Cardiac enlargement or failure.
• Pericardial effusion.
• ECG changes of pericarditis, myocarditis, AV block, or other cardiac arrythmias.

SUMMARY PLAN FOR EXAMINATION OF THE CARDIOVASCULAR SYSTEM

General
Breathing pattern
Cyanosis
Anaemia
Oedema
Arteries and veins
Pulse – rate, rhythm, volume, character
Blood pressure
Jugular venous pulse and pressure
Peripheral pulses
Arterial bruits
The heart
Inspection
Palpation
  Apex beat
  Parasternal heave
  Thrills
Auscultation
  Heart sounds
  Murmurs
  Pericardial friction rub.

CLINICAL SIGNS OF COMMON CARDIAC PROBLEMS

Now that you are familiar with the symptoms and signs of disease of the cardiovascular system describe the clinical signs which you would expect to find in the conditions outlined below. Proceed in order of inspection, palpation and auscultation, ensuring that you understand the origin of the signs.

Q1.139 What are the clinical signs of mitral stenosis?

A:
- Mitral facies or malar flush.[1]
- Pulse, small volume and often atrial fibrillation.
- Apex beat displaced downwards and tapping in character.
- Diastolic thrill may be palpable at apex.
- Left parasternal heave.
- Loud and often palpable first sound at apex, and possibly loud second sound in the pulmonary area due to pulmonary hypertension.
- An opening snap.
- A low-pitched, rumbling, mid-diastolic murmur best heard at the apex, or just internal to the apex.[2] The murmur may show presystolic accentuation if the patient is in sinus rhythm. It is not conducted, and may be most clearly heard with the patient lying on the left side.

1. Seen in severe mitral stenosis with pulmonary hypertension.
2. In some cases of mitral stenosis there may be no diastolic murmur audible because of a reduction in cardiac output and resultant reduction in flow across mitral valve. The first heart sound, however, is usually increased and there is an opening snap.

Q1.140 What are the clinical signs of mitral regurgitation?

A:
- Pulse usually unremarkable.
- Apex beat displaced laterally and thrusting in character.
- A systolic thrill may be palpable.
- First heart sound at the apex may be diminished or soft.
- A prominent third heart sound.[1]
- A pansystolic murmur best heard at the apex but which radiates laterally to the axilla and back.

1. Caused by sudden rush of blood back into the dilated left ventricle in early diastole.

Q1.141 What are the clinical signs of aortic stenosis?

A: • Pulse is slow rising/slow falling, i.e. anacrotic or plateau pulse.
• Apex beat is displaced laterally and is heaving in character.[1]
• The second heart sound in the aortic area is diminished or absent.
• Reversed splitting of the second heart sound.
• A rough, mid-systolic murmur best heard in the aortic area and upper right sternal border. It may be associated with a thrill and is conducted into the neck and towards the apex.

1. Cardiomegaly may not be obvious clinically.

Q1.142 What are the clinical signs of aortic regurgitation?

A: • Collapsing pulse.
• Capillary pulsation in the nail bed.
• Marked carotid pulsation (Corrigan's sign).[1]
• Femoral systolic bruit or femoral 'pistol shots'.
• Wide pulse pressure.
• Apex beat displaced laterally and downwards, and thrusting in character.
• A high-pitched, blowing, early diastolic murmur best heard along the left sternal edge with the diaphragm of the stethoscope and with the patient sitting up, leaning forward, and holding the breath in expiration.
• An Austin Flint murmur.

1. Other high output states may also be associated with increased carotid pulsation. The carotid pulse is also visible when the carotid artery is kinked or aneurysmal.

Q1.143 What are the clinical signs of tricuspid stenosis?[1]

A:
- Prominent jugular venous 'a' wave.
- Low-pitched, rumbling, diastolic murmur best heard at the lower right or left sternal edge, and which is louder on inspiration.
- Hepatomegaly, ascites and oedema may be present.

1. An uncommon valve lesion, due mainly to rheumatic heart disease. Also associated with carcinoid syndrome.

Q1.144 What are the clinical signs of tricuspid regurgitation?[1]

A:
- Atrial fibrillation common.
- Prominent jugular venous 'v' wave.
- Blowing pansystolic murmur, best heard at the lower right or left sternal edge on inspiration.
- Palpable pulsatile liver.
- Ascites and dependent oedema may be present.

1. May be functional following right ventricular dilatation. Other causes include rheumatic heart disease, infective endocarditis, carcinoid syndrome and Ebstein's anomaly (congenital malposition of the tricuspid valve).

Q1.145 What are the clinical signs of pulmonary stenosis?[1]

A:
- Low volume pulse.
- Prominent jugular venous 'a' wave may be visible.
- Left parasternal heave.
- Systolic thrill.
- Pulmonary second sound diminished or absent.
- Harsh mid-systolic murmur heard in the pulmonary area.

1. Usually congenital; rarely due to rheumatic heart disease and the carcinoid syndrome.

Q1.146 What clinical signs may be seen in pulmonary hypertension from any cause?

A: • Low volume pulse.
• Prominent 'a' wave in jugular venous pulse.
• Parasternal (right ventricular) heave.
• Loud pulmonary second sound.
• Right ventricular fourth heart sound.
• An early mid-diastolic murmur.[1]
• Pansystolic murmur and prominent 'v' wave in jugular venous pulse.[2]

1. Graham Steell murmur due to functional pulmonary regurgitation found in severe pulmonary hypertension.
2. Signs of tricuspid regurgitation.

Q1.147 What clinical signs may be found in hypertrophic cardiomyopathy (HCM)?

A: • Jerky carotid pulse.[1]
• Ejection systolic murmur which may be 'late', i.e. continuing until the second sound.
• Pansystolic murmur due to mitral regurgitation.
• Loud fourth heart sound.[2]

1. Due to abnormal left ventricular outflow.
2. Due to mitral regurgitation and/or 'stiffness' of ventricle.

Q1.148 What are the common clinical signs of a restrictive cardiomyopathy?

A: • Elevated jugular venous pressure with diastolic collapse (Freidreich's sign).
• Elevation of jugular venous pressure on inspiration (Kussmaul's sign).
• Cardiac enlargement.
• Hepatomegaly.
• Ascites.
• Leg oedema.

Q1.149 What are the common signs of pericardial effusion?

A:
- Elevated jugular pressure with diastolic collapse (Freidreich's sign).
- Elevation of jugular venous pressure on inspiration (Kussmaul's sign).
- Pulsus paradoxus.
- Apex beat may not be palpable.
- Heart sounds soft.

Q1.150 What are the common signs of constrictive pericarditis?

A:
- Signs of pericardial effusion.
- Hepatomegaly.
- Ascites.
- Dependent oedema.

Q1.151 What signs may be seen in congenital heart disease irrespective of the cause?

A:
- Central cyanosis.[1]
- Pulmonary hypertension.[2]
- Clubbing of fingers.
- Paradoxical embolism.[3]
- Retarded growth.
- Syncope.[4]
- Squatting.[5]

1. Will be seen, for example, in ventricular septal defect if shunting of blood changes from left-to-right to right-to-left (i.e. pulmonary arterial pressure equals systemic pressure – Eisenmenger's syndrome).
2. Results from large left-to-right shunting of blood.
3. May occur through communication between right and left heart.
4. Common if severe pulmonary or aortic stenosis.
5. Posture adopted by children with Fallot's tetralogy.

Q1.152 What are the clinical signs of atrial septal defect (ASD)?

A:
- Right ventricular heave.
- Fixed splitting of the second sound.
- Mid-systolic murmur best heard in the pulmonary area and the left sternal edge.[1]
- Mid-diastolic murmur best heard at the lower end of the sternum.[2]

1. Due to increased blood flow through the pulmonary valve.
2. A functional tricuspid flow murmur.

Q1.153 What are the clinical signs of a moderate or severe ventricular septal defect (VSD)?

A:
- No cyanosis unless right-to-left shunt.
- Apex beat displaced laterally and heaving in character.
- Palpable systolic thrill at lower left sternal edge.
- Parasternal heave and a loud pulmonary second sound may be present.
- Rough pansystolic murmur at left sternal edge and apex.
- Mid-diastolic murmur at apex if septal defect severe.[1]

1. Due to increased flow through the mitral valve.

Q1.154 What cardiac lesions are found in Fallot's tetralogy?

A:
- A ventricular septal defect.
- Right ventricular outflow obstruction, i.e. pulmonary stenosis.
- An 'overriding' aorta above the ventricular septal defect.
- Right ventricular hypertrophy.

Q1.155 What are the common clinical features of Fallot's tetralogy?

A:
- Finger clubbing.
- Central cyanosis.
- Squatting posture.

- Parasternal heave.
- Mid-systolic ejection murmur loudest in the pulmonary area.
- Palpable thrill.

Q1.156 What are the clinical signs of patent ductus arteriosus?

A:
- Large volume, bounding pulse.
- Wide pulse pressure.
- Apex beat heaving in character.
- Palpable thrill may be felt.
- Continuous 'machinery' murmur best heard in the pulmonary area and below left clavicle, and which radiates to the back.

Q1.157 What are the major clinical features of coarctation of the aorta?

A:
- Visible and/or palpable collateral vessels on the back of the chest.
- Weak and delayed femoral pulses.
- Hypertension in upper limbs.
- Left ventricular hypertrophy.
- Mid-to-late systolic murmur over upper precordium or back.
- Vascular bruits in collateral circulation.
- There may be evidence of aortic stenosis.[1]

1. Eighty per cent of patients have a bicuspid aortic valve which may be stenotic.

2
THE RESPIRATORY SYSTEM

HISTORY AND SYMPTOMS OF LUNG DISEASE

Q2.1 What are the six most important symptoms of respiratory disease?

A: 1. Cough.
2. Sputum.
3. Haemoptysis.
4. Breathlessness.
5. Wheeze.
6. Chest pain.

Q2.2 Name other specific symptoms of disease of the upper respiratory tract

A: • Hoarseness and loss of voice.[1]
• Nasal discharge.[2]
• Nasal blockage.
• Sneezing.
• Nose bleeds (epistaxis).[3]

1. May be due, for example, to laryngitis or infiltration of recurrent laryngeal nerves by tumour.
2. May be profuse or watery as in rhinitis, or thick and mucopurulent in latter stages of the common cold or in acute or chronic sinusitis.
3. It is usually easy to distinguish between epistaxis and haemoptysis. However, if bleeding occurs in the more posterior parts of the nasal cavity, it may be inhaled and, when coughed up, thought to come from the lungs.

Q2.3 What important non- specific symptoms may be found in patients with respiratory infections?

A: • Loss of appetite and weight.[1]
    • Sweating.[2]
    • Joint pains and myalgia.[2]
    • Headache and other neurological symptoms.[2]
    • Gastrointestinal symptoms including vomiting and diarrhoea.[2]

1. Weight loss and nocturnal sweating are common in tuberculosis.
2. Some or all of these symptoms may be associated with lung infection due to *Mycoplasma pneumoniae*, *Chlamydia psittaci*, *Legionella pneumophila* and *Coxiella burnetii*. Diarrhoea may also be seen in patients with *Pneumocystis carinii* infection. In pneumonias due to these organisms systemic symptoms may overshadow respiratory symptoms. Joint diseases, such as rheumatoid arthritis may be associated with pulmonary complications (page 146, Q8.18).

COUGH

Q2.4 In a patient with chronic cough what should you ask about the cough?

A: • Duration.
    • Progression.[1]
    • When worse.[2]
    • Precipitating factors.[3]
    • Is it productive?
    • Association with pain.
    • Association with haemoptysis.

1. A progressively worsening cough in the Western world should alert one to the possibility of bronchial carcinoma and, in the developing world, of tuberculosis.
2. Nocturnal cough is common in asthma and pulmonary oedema.
3. Cigarette smoke, dust, cold air, foggy weather.

Q2.5 What diagnoses should you consider in patients with chronic cough?

A:
- Smoking.
- Chronic bronchitis.[1]
- Tuberculosis.
- Asthma.[2]
- Lung cancer.
- Postviral infection.
- Postnasal drip.
- Bronchiectasis.

1. The diagnosis of chronic bronchitis is diagnosed on the patient's history and is defined as the presence of a productive cough on most days for at least 3 months of the year for more than one year.
2. Cough may be the predominant symptom of asthma, especially in children.

SPUTUM

Q2.6 Sputum production is always abnormal. What should you ask about the sputum?

A:
- Quantity.
- Colour and variation in the colour.[1]
- When most profuse.
- Smell.[2]

1. Clear white and mucoid in chronic bronchitis. A green or yellow colour usually indicates infection. A rusty colour may be seen in pneumonia, a pinkish colour in pulmonary oedema and, very rarely, chocolate-coloured in klebsiella pneumonia and ruptured amoebic abscess. The colour of the sputum may vary, e.g. in chronic bronchitis when bacterial infection supervenes.
2. A foul smell suggests an anaerobic infection.

HAEMOPTYSIS

Q2.7 What are important causes of haemoptysis?

A:
- Acute infections, e.g. lobar pneumonia.
- Tuberculosis.[1]

- Bronchial carcinoma.[1]
- Bronchiectasis.[1]
- Lung abscess.[1]
- Pulmonary hypertension, e.g. secondary to mitral stenosis.
- Pulmonary infarction.
- Trauma.[2]
- Mycetoma.[1,2]
- Goodpasture's syndrome.[2]
- Idiopathic pulmonary haemosiderosis.[2]
- Blood disorders.[2]
- Benign tumours.[2]

1. May be associated with massive haemoptysis.
2. Rare causes of haemoptysis.

BREATHLESSNESS

Q2.8 What points should be noted about breathlessness?

A:
- Experienced at rest, or when lying flat[1] or only on exercise.[2]
- Precipitating factors.[3]
- Episodic.[4]
- Worse at particular time of day.[5]
- Associated with chest pain.

1. In left ventricular failure and severe airway obstruction, breathlessness is worse on lying flat (orthopnoea).
2. Ask how far patient can walk. Can he dress without feeling breathless?
3. Emotion, change of environment, dust, etc.
4. Typical of asthma.
5. Asthmatic symptoms may initially be worse at night.

Q2.9 What are the characteristics of breathlessness which might suggest the diagnosis of asthma?

A:
- Associated with wheezing.
- Commonly associated with cough.
- Breathlessness is episodic.
- May be worse after prolonged exercise.

- May be worse at night.
- Attacks of breathlessness may be precipitated by inhalation of dry cold air, irritant dust, cigarette smoke, allergens, emotion, etc.

WHEEZE

Q2.10 Which patients commonly complain of wheeze?

A: Patients with asthma or chronic bronchitis and emphysema, but wheeze may also occur in patients with left heart failure.

Q2.11 With what can the wheeze of asthma or bronchitis be confused if you fail to examine patient carefully?

A: Inspiratory wheeze or stridor due to narrowing of larynx or trachea.

CHEST PAIN

Q2.12 What features of chest pain due to respiratory disease should be noted?

A: • Location.[1]
   • Character.[2]
   • Affected by respiration, cough, movement or exercise.[3]

1. The pain of tracheitis is central whilst pleuritic pain is lateral. Inflammation of the central part of the diaphragm may lead to pain in the shoulder, whilst inflammation of lateral part of the diaphragm may be associated with pain in lower lateral chest wall and upper abdomen.
2. Pleuritic pain is sharp or stabbing.
3. Pleuritic pain is typically made worse by coughing, respiration or movement.

Q2.13 What are common pulmonary causes of pleuritic chest pain?

A: • Pneumonia.

- Tuberculosis.
- Lung abscess.
- Pulmonary infarction.
- Malignancy.
- Pneumothorax.

Q2.14 Pain arising from the chest wall may also cause pleuritic-like pain. Give examples of common problems affecting chest wall structures

A:
- Fractured ribs.
- Herpes zoster.[1]
- Root pain associated with spinal disease.
- Local pain and tenderness of muscles or costal cartilages due to Coxsackie B virus.

1. Pain may be felt before rash appears.

PAST MEDICAL HISTORY

Q2.15 What conditions should be looked for in the past medical history?

A:
- Tuberculosis including BCG vaccination.
- Childhood chest illnesses.[1]
- Recent trauma.
- Recent operation.[2]
- Allergic disorders.[3]
- Diabetes mellitus.[4]

1. May lead to development of bronchiectasis.
2. Operations may be complicated by deep venous thrombosis and pulmonary thromboembolism.
3. Hay fever, eczema.
4. Patients with diabetes in developing countries have a greatly increased risk of tuberculosis. Any diabetic patient complaining of chronic cough should have a chest radiograph and sputum checked for acid-fast bacilli.

SOCIAL/FAMILY/DRUG HISTORY

Q2.16 In the social history what points should be noted?

A:
- Smoking.[1]
- Alcohol.[2]
- Occupation including work and contact with asbestos.[3]
- Contact with animals.
- Travel abroad.[4]

1. Enquire about number of cigarettes smoked and duration of smoking.
2. Heavy drinkers have an increased risk of tuberculosis.
3. Do not ask only about present occupation. Patient may have had a job in the past which involved exposure to industrial dusts.
4. May be of relevance, for example, in patients with simple and prolonged pulmonary eosinophilia, and tropical pulmonary eosinophilia.

Q2.17 What drugs may be associated with wheeze?

A:
- Aspirin.
- NSAIDS.
- Non-selective, β-adrenoceptor-blocking drugs (e.g. propranolol).
- Penicillins.[1]
- Sulphonamides.[1]
- Cephalosporins.[1]

1. Rare.

Q2.18 Is family history of value in patients with lung disease?

A: Yes, for example, patients with extrinsic or atopic asthma may have an affected relative with asthma, eczema or hay fever and patients with tuberculosis may have close family contact.

EXAMINATION

CHEST EXAMINATION

Q2.19 Does careful examination of the chest really matter if a chest radiograph is available?

A: Yes – clinical examination may reveal severe disease despite a normal chest radiograph, e.g. asthma. It is also much more useful in assessing pathophysiology. A chest radiograph cannot therefore be regarded as an adequate substitute for clinical examination.

Q2.20 Is a basic knowledge of anatomy of value in examination of the chest?

A: It is essential in the localization and description of abnormal findings. It is also necessary in the performance of practical procedures such as aspiration of pleural fluid.

Q2.21 In describing the site of abnormal signs which two methods can you use?

A: 1. Abnormal findings may be localized anatomically, e.g. apex of right upper lobe, base of left lower lobe, right middle lobe, etc.
   2. Abnormal findings may be described according to zones, i.e. upper, middle, and lower zones anteriorly, posteriorly and laterally. This method is probably best.

Q2.22 What are surface markings of the oblique fissure?

A: The oblique fissure runs from the lower end of the fourth thoracic vertebrae (posterior end of the fifth rib) to the sixth rib in the mid-clavicular line (sixth costochondral junction) and on to the diaphragm anteriorly.

Q2.23 What are surface markings of the transverse fissure?

A: The transverse fissure runs horizontally from the fourth rib anteriorly on the right to meet the oblique fissure in the mid-axillary line.

Q2.24 What is best way of numbering the ribs anteriorly?

A: By identification of the second rib at the manubriosternal angle.

Q2.25 Before you begin to examine the chest what clinical features should be looked for outside the chest?

A: • Clubbing of fingers.
   • Nicotine stains.
   • Cyanosis – peripheral and central.
   • Clinical signs of raised PCO_2 (hypercapnia).
   • Pulsus paradoxus.[1]
   • Raised jugular venous pressure.[2]
   • Cervical and axillary lymphadenopathy.

   1. May be present in severe acute asthma.
   2. Due to cor pulmonale

CLUBBING

Q2.26 What are the five stages of clubbing?

A: i.   Increased nail bed fluctuation.
   ii. Loss of angle between nail and nail bed.[1]
   iii. Increased curvature of long and transverse axes of nail.
   iv. Increased bulk of soft tissues at the ends of the fingers.
   v.   Hypertrophic pulmonary osteoarthropathy.[2]

   1. Normally $140°$.
   2. Rare – arthralgia with joint swelling of wrists and ankles occurs. Radiograph shows subperiosteal new bone formation. Bronchogenic carcinoma is the most common association.

Q2.27 What are causes of clubbing?

A: 1. Respiratory disease:
- Bronchiectasis.
- Lung abscess.
- Empyema.
- Bronchial carcinoma.
- Mesothelioma.
- Fibrosing alveolitis.
- Asbestosis.
- Cystic fibrosis.

2. Non-respiratory disease:
- Infective endocarditis.
- Cyanotic congenital heart disease.
- Hepatic cirrhosis.
- Ulcerative colitis.
- Crohn's disease.
- Pyelonephritis.
- Coeliac disease.
- Congenital.

CYANOSIS

Q2.28 What is the cause of cyanosis?

A: Cyanosis is due to an excess of reduced circulating haemoglobin, i.e. hypoxia. Traditionally, at least 5 g dl^{-1} of haemoglobin must be present before cyanosis is apparent, but recent studies have shown that 1.5 g dl^{-1} is enough. (Cyanosis may also be rarely due to the presence of other reduction products of haemoglobin such as sulphaemoglobin or methaemoglobin.)

Q2.29 How is cyanosis classified?

A: Into peripheral and central cyanosis.

Q2.30 What causes peripheral cyanosis?

A: Peripheral cyanosis is associated with:

- A low cardiac output as in congestive heart failure or shock.
- Peripheral vascular disease.
- Exposure to cold.

It is detected by examination of fingers and nails. Blue lips are also a sign of peripheral cyanosis. Hands are normally cold. If they are warm and cyanosed, the cyanosis may reflect central cyanosis.

Q2.31 What causes central cyanosis?

A: Central cyanosis is usually due to lung diseases such as chronic bronchitis and severe pulmonary fibrosis where there is inadequate oxygenation of the blood. It is also seen in heart failure, pulmonary embolism and in cardiac disease where there is a right-to-left intracardiac shunt.

Q2.32 Where is central cyanosis best detected?

A: Tongue and buccal mucosa.

Q2.33 What are the signs of carbon dioxide retention?

A: • Flapping tremor.
    • Peripheral venous dilatation.
    • Bounding pulse.
    • Warm extremities.
    • Confusion and drowsiness.
    • Papilloedema.

JUGULAR VENOUS PRESSURE

Q2.34 What pulmonary conditions are associated with a raised jugular venous pressure?

A: • Cor pulmonale.[1]
    • Superior vena caval obstruction due usually to malignant disease.

    1. Right heart failure due to chronic lung diseases such as chronic bronchitis and emphysema.

INSPECTION OF CHEST

Q2.35 What features should be noted on inspection?

A: • Respiratory rate.[1]
    • Breathing pattern.
    • Deformity of chest.
    • Chest wall movements.[2]
    • Indrawing of intercostal spaces.[3]

- Use of accessory muscles.
- Prominent veins on chest.[4]

1. Normally 14–20 breaths per minute.
2. May be asymmetrical in patients with pneumothorax, pleural effusion, unilateral pulmonary fibrosis, etc.
3. Usually associated with chronic airflow limitation.
4. May indicate obstruction of the superior vena cava.

Q2.36 What abnormalities in breathing patterns may be commonly seen?

A:
- Rapid and shallow breathing in patients with weak respiratory muscles, stiff lungs or pleurisy.
- Rapid, deep breathing in metabolic acidosis due to diabetic ketoacidosis, or salicylate poisoning.
- Prolonged expiratory phase in patients with airflow obstruction.
- Alternating periods of apnoea and hyperpnoea (Cheyne–Stokes respiration) in patients with severe cerebral disease, e.g. stroke or left ventricular failure.

Q2.37 What deformities of the chest are commonly seen in patients with chest disease?

A:
- Kyphoscoliosis.
- Hyperinflation in emphysema (barrel chest).
- Flattening and diminished movement of one side of chest due, for example, to underlying collapse.

PALPATION OF CHEST

Q2.38 What five things should always be checked when palpating the chest?

A:
- Position of the trachea and apex for evidence of mediastinal shift.
- Assessment of extent and symmetry of respiratory movements.[1]
- Tactile vocal fremitus.[2]
- Lymph nodes.[3]
- Breasts in females.[4]

1. Chest expansion should be at least 5 cm.
2. Tactile vocal fremitus provides information similar to that provided by vocal resonance. Some clinicians consider that tactile vocal resonance should be discarded and only vocal resonance performed.
3. Look for lymph nodes in neck, supraclavicular fossae and axillae.
4. Pendulous breasts may conceal a carcinoma which has spread to lymph nodes or metastasized to lung.

Q2.39 What lung disease may cause mediastinal shift?

A: • A pleural effusion or pneumothorax may push the mediastinum away from the affected side of the chest.
  • Pulmonary fibrosis and lung collapse (atelectasis) may pull the mediastinum towards the affected side of the chest.

Q2.40 What pathologies are associated with an increase in tactile vocal fremitus?

A: • Consolidation as in lobar pneumonia.
  • Cavitation (sometimes).

Q2.41 What pathologies are associated with a decrease in tactile vocal fremitus?

A: • Pleural effusion.
  • Large pneumothorax.
  • Collapse (atelectasis).

Percussion

Q2.42 What conditions are associated with a loss of cardiac dullness?

A: • Emphysema.
  • Pneumothorax.

Q2.43 What conditions are commonly associated with hyperresonance?

A: • Emphysema.
  • Pneumothorax.[1]

1. Often very difficult to detect.

Q2.44 What conditions are associated with dullness on percussion?

A: • Pleural effusion.[1]
• Pleural thickening.
• Consolidation.
• Atelectasis.
• Lung abscess.[2]

1. Dullness 'stony'.
2. Rarely found in developed countries.

Q2.45 In a normal supine subject what is the upper level of liver dullness?

A: At the sixth rib in the mid-clavicular line.

Q2.46 How do you distinguish between a pleural effusion and raised diaphragm as causes of basal dullness?

A: Ask the patient to inspire. If dullness is due to a raised diaphragm the dullness will move downwards if the diaphragm is not paralysed.

AUSCULTATION

Q2.47 What three things do you listen for on auscultation?

A: 1. Breath sounds:
   (a) whether vesicular or bronchial;
   (b) whether vesicular breath sounds altered in intensity.*
2. Voice sounds, i.e. vocal resonance, and whispering pectoriloquy.
3. Added sounds.

* Sometimes the term 'diminished air entry' is used when breath sounds are diminished in intensity. It is better, however, to speak of diminished breath sounds, i.e. what you hear, since diminished breath sounds may not always be due to reduced air entry.

Q2.48 What conditions are associated with diminished breath sounds?

A:
- Thick chest wall.
- Emphysema.
- Pneumothorax.
- Pleural effusion or pleural thickening.
- Atelectasis.
- Fibrosis.[1]

1. Not always associated with diminished breath sounds.

Q2.49 What conditions are associated with bronchial breathing?

A:
- Consolidation.
- Cavitation.[1]
- Above a pleural effusion.[2]
- Over collapsed lung.

1. Rarely heard in developed countries but common in developing countries.
2. Rarely heard. Consolidation and cavitation are by far the most important conditions associated with bronchial breathing.

Q2.50 What conditions are associated with increased vocal resonance?

A:
- Consolidation.
- Cavitation.

Q2.51 In what conditions will vocal resonance be diminished?

A: Those in which breath sounds are diminished or absent (see Q2.48).

Q2.52 What are the three main added sounds which may be heard?

A: 1. Wheezes (ronchi).*

2. Crackles (crepitations).
3. Pleural friction rub.

* Here wheeze is a sign, not a symptom, i.e. a sign usually of obstructive airways disease.

Q2.53 How are crackles (crepitations) classified?

A: • As fine[1] or coarse.[2]
   • Early inspiratory[3] or late inspiratory.[4]

1. Fine in early pneumonia or pulmonary oedema.
2. Coarse in bronchiectasis or pulmonary fibrosis.
3. Early inspiratory in airflow limitation.
4. Late inspiratory in pulmonary oedema and pulmonary fibrosis.

SUMMARY OF STEPS IN EXAMINATION OF THE RESPIRATORY SYSTEM

Examination of the chest should be carried out in the following order.

1. Inspection:
   (a) cyanosis
   (b) jugular venous pressure
   (c) respiratory rate
   (d) breathing patterns
   (e) any deformity of chest
   (f) chest wall movements
   (g) indrawing of intercostal muscles
   (h) use of accessory muscles
2. Palpation:
   (a) trachea and apex
   (b) extent and symmetry of respiratory movements
   (c) tactile vocal fremitus
   (d) lymph nodes
   (e) breasts
3. Percussion.
4. Auscultation.
   (a) breath sounds:
       (i) vesicular or bronchial
       (ii) vesicular breath sounds diminished or absent
   (b) voice sounds, i.e. vocal resonance
   (c) Added sounds:
       (i) wheezes (ronchi)
       (ii) crackles (crepitations)
       (iii) pleural friction rub.

CLINICAL SIGNS OF COMMON CHEST PROBLEMS

Now that you are familiar with the method of examining the chest, how well can you describe the abnormal findings which you would expect in the conditions below? Describe your findings in the usual order of inspection, palpation, percussion, auscultation.

Q2.54 What are the clinical signs of a pleural effusion?

A:
- Respiratory rate increased if effusion large.
- Chest movement diminished on side of effusion.
- Trachea and apex may be shifted away from the side of the effusion.
- Tactile vocal fremitus absent.
- Percussion note 'stony' dull.
- Breath sounds absent or greatly diminished.
- Bronchial breathing may be heard above the level of effusion as well as aegophony.[1]
- Vocal resonance decreased.
- No added sounds.

1. Aegophony refers to nasal or bleating quality of voice above the level of a pleural effusion.

Q2.55 What are the clinical signs of lobar pneumonia?

A:
- Respiratory rate increased.
- Patient's breathing rapid and shallow.
- Reduced movement on the affected side may be observed.
- Trachea and apex will not be displaced.
- Tactile vocal fremitus increased.
- Percussion note dull over area of consolidation.
- Vocal resonance increased with whispering pectoriloquy.
- Bronchial breathing.
- Pleural friction rub may be audible.
- Crackles audible during stage of resolution.

Q2.56 What are the clinical signs of a large pneumothorax?

A:
- Respiratory rate increased.
- Reduced movement of chest wall on side of lesion.
- Trachea and apex may be shifted away from side of lesion.
- Tactile vocal fremitus absent or diminished.
- Percussion note hyperresonant.[1]
- Breath sounds absent or diminished over affected side.
- Vocal resonance absent or diminished.
- No added sounds.

1. By no means always detectable.

Q2.57 What are the clinical signs of severe bronchial asthma?

A:
- Expiratory phase prolonged, patient too breathless to speak.
- Indrawing of intercostal muscles.
- Accessory muscles in use.
- Chest expansion symmetrical but diminished.
- Percussion note normal.
- Breath sounds vesicular with prolonged expiratory phase.[1]
- Widespread wheezes.

1. If breath sounds are not audible this indicates severe airway obstruction requiring very urgent action.

Q2.58 What are the clinical signs of massive atelectasis or collapse of the right lung?

A:
- Respiratory rate increased.
- Chest wall movements asymmetrical with diminished movement on affected side.
- Trachea and apex shifted towards right side.
- Tactile vocal fremitus absent or diminished over affected side.
- Percussion note dull.
- Clinical evidence of elevation of right dome of diaphragm.

- Breath sounds absent or diminished on affected side.
- Compensatory emphysema of left lung may be found.
- Vocal resonance reduced or absent.
- No added sounds.

Q2.59 What are the clinical signs of chronic bronchitis and emphysema?

A: • Chest wall movements limited on both sides.
- Barrel-shaped chest – lungs hyperinflated.
- Patient tachypnoeic with prolonged expiration.
- Accessory muscles of respiration in use.
- Indrawing on inspiration of suprasternal and supra-clavicular notches, as well as intercostal muscles.
- Apex beat may be difficult to palpate.
- Trachea central.
- Percussion note normal or hyperresonant with loss of normal cardiac and liver dullness.
- Breath sounds may be diminished over both lungs.
- Crackles and expiratory wheezes may be audible.

Q2.60 What are the clinical signs of cryptogenic fibrosing alveolitis?

A: • Respiratory rate increased.
- Chest wall movement diminished on both sides.
- Accessory muscles in use.
- Trachea and apex central.
- Percussion note normal.
- Breath sounds normal vesicular.
- Vocal resonance may be increased.
- Widespread crackles.

Q2.61 What are the clinical signs of fibrosis localized to the right upper lobe?

A: • Chest wall movement may be diminished over area of right upper lobe.
- Flattening of chest wall over the same area.
- Trachea may be deviated to the right.
- Percussion note may be dull over the right upper lobe anteriorly.

- Breath sounds normal vesicular or bronchial.
- Vocal resonance may be normal or increased.
- Crackles audible over right upper lobe.

Q2.62 What are the clinical signs of acute left ventricular failure?

A:
- Respiratory rate increased, patient may be gasping for breath.
- Tachycardia.
- Elevated jugular venous pressure may be seen.
- Apex may be displaced as a result of cardiomegaly.
- Percussion note may be dull, particularly over both lower lobes.
- Gallop rhythm.
- Breath sounds normal vesicular.
- Crackles audible throughout the lungs, especially in lower lobes.
- Wheezes may also be audible.
- Signs of pleural effusion may be detected.

Q2.63 What are the clinical signs of cavitation in the right upper lobe?

A:
- There may be no abnormality on inspection.
- Trachea central.
- Tactile vocal fremitus may be increased.
- Percussion note may be normal or dull.
- Bronchial breathing may be audible.
- Vocal resonance may be increased.
- Crackles may be audible.

Q2.64 Pleural fluid may be a transudate or exudate. How is an exudate distinguished from a transudate?

A: An exudate has a protein content greater than 30 g/l and the lactic dehydrogenase is greater than 200 IU/l, whilst a transudate has a protein content of less than 30 g/l and the lactic dehydrogenase is less than 200 IU/l.

Q2.65 What are some of the common and not-so-common causes of an exudate?

A:
- Bacterial pneumonia.
- Carcinoma of bronchus.
- Tuberculosis.
- Pulmonary infarction.
- Connective tissue disease.
- Postmyocardial infarction syndrome.[1]
- Acute pancreatitis.[1]
- Mesothelioma.[1]
- Sarcoidosis.[1]
- Familial Mediterranean fever.[1]

1. Rare causes of an exudative pleural effusion.

Q2.66 What are some of the common and less common causes of a transudate?

A:
- Heart failure.
- Hypoproteinaemia (e.g. nephrotic syndrome).
- Constrictive pericarditis.
- Hypothyroidism.
- Meigs' syndrome.[1]

1. Ovarian tumour associated with right-sided pleural effusion.

3
THE ALIMENTARY SYSTEM AND LIVER

SYMPTOMS OF DISEASES OF THE ALIMENTARY TRACT AND THE LIVER

Q3.1 What are the important symptoms of disease of the alimentary tract?

A:
- Abdominal pain.
- Difficulty in swallowing (dysphagia).
- Vomiting.
- Weight loss.
- Change in bowel habit.
- Swelling of abdomen.
- Tenesmus.
- Diarrhoea.
- Rectal bleeding.
- Jaundice.

Q3.2 Name other symptoms encountered in patients with alimentary disease, but which may be of variable significance in terms of underlying organic disease

A:
- Anorexia.[1]
- Nausea.[2]
- Flatus.[3]
- Belching.[4]
- Reflux and water-brash.[5]
- Heartburn.[6]
- Constipation.[7]

1. Anorexia occurs in many conditions including alimentary diseases. It is also a common symptom of viral hepatitis.
2. May be a symptom of a wide variety of problems outside the gastrointestinal tract, e.g. pregnancy, uraemia, migraine, drug ingestion, etc.
3. Refers to passage of gas rectally.
4. Very rarely is this a symptom of organic disease.
5. Regurgitation of bitter fluid into the mouth.
6. A burning sensation in the epigastrium and behind the sternum. A common symptom of peptic ulceration. If related to posture it suggests gastro-oesophageal reflux.
7. Important to know what the patient means by constipation. Generally patients attach undue significance to any decrease in the frequency of passage of stool.

ABDOMINAL PAIN

Q3.3 Abdominal pain is a very important symptom of alimentary disease. What features should be noted about the pain?

A: • Duration.
   • Character.[1]
   • Site.[2]
   • Radiation.[3]
   • Periodicity.[4]
   • Whether felt at special times.[5]
   • Aggravating and relieving factors.[6]
   • Association with micturition or periods (dysuria, dysmenorrhoea).
   • Association with fever and urethral discharge.[7]
   • Association with pain in other systems.[8]

1. The patient may use many different adjectives to describe the pain.
2. May be localized or diffuse. The pain of peptic ulcer may not always be localized to the epigastrium.
3. The pain of renal colic may radiate to the groins and genitalia, and the pain of peptic ulcer may radiate to the back.

4. The pain of peptic ulcer is typically episodic with periods of freedom from pain lasting for days or months.
5. Nocturnal pain or pain between meals is typical of peptic ulcer.
6. Peptic ulcer pain is often relieved by food, milk and antacids, and may be aggravated by irregular meals and smoking. Alcohol may aggravate acute pancreatitis, and the pain of acute pancreatitis may be relieved by sitting upright.
7. Consider the possibility of septic abortion and pelvic inflammatory disease.
8. Many patients, especially at outpatient clinics, complain also of pain in other systems. If symptoms are difficult to fit together into any kind of diagnostic pattern consider the possibility of a psychosomatic problem.

Q3.4 Does abdominal pain always indicate a problem in the alimentary and genitourinary tract?

A: No, pain may arise from structures outside the abdomen, and from infectious and metabolic problems.

Q3.5 Name several extra-abdominal problems which may present with or be associated with abdominal pain. How may they be classified?

A: • Problems arising from the chest:
    (a) pleurisy;
    (b) myocardial infarction.
• Metabolic and endocrine problems:
    (a) severe diabetic ketoacidosis;[1]
    (b) hypercalcaemia;[2]
    (c) acute intermittent porphyria;[2]
    (d) Addison's disease.[2]
• Neurological problems:
    (a) compression of nerve roots;
    (b) herpes zoster.[3]

1. Urine should be tested for glucose and ketones in every patient presenting as an emergency with abdominal pain.

2. Rare.
3. Pain may precede appearance of the rash.

Q3.6 What are common 'surgical' causes of acute abdominal pain in adults?

A:
- Acute peritonitis.
- Intestinal obstruction.
- Acute appendicitis.
- Acute cholecystitis.
- Renal colic.
- Diverticulitis.
- Pain arising from pelvic organs in females, e.g. ruptured ectopic pregnancy.
- Acute obstruction of superior mesenteric artery.

Q3.7 What are the main medical intra-abdominal problems which may present with acute abdominal pain?

A:
- Acute pancreatitis.
- Acute pyelonephritis.[1]
- Peptic ulceration.
- Bowel ischaemia due to sickle-cell disease or to Henoch–Schönlein syndrome.
- Gastroenteritis.[2]
- Congestion of liver.[3]
- Constipation.[4]

1. Pain usually felt in loins but sometimes in bladder area.
2. There will usually be associated diarrhoea and/or vomiting.
   Worm infestation may also cause abdominal pain.
3. In acute hepatitis or congestive cardiac failure, but pain is rarely acute.
4. In the elderly, constipation may cause severe abdominal pain.

DYSPHAGIA

Q3.8 Why is dysphagia such an important symptom?

A: It frequently indicates cancer of the oesophagus.

Q3.9 What points should be asked about dysphagia?

A: • Duration.
    • Progression.
    • Worse with liquids or solids, or both.
    • Association with heartburn.
    • Association with painful mouth or painful swallowing.[1]

    1. May indicate oesophageal candidiasis. Look for evidence of oral thrush.

VOMITING

Q3.10 Are nausea and vomiting always symptoms of alimentary disease?

A: No, nausea and vomiting may be associated with a wide variety of problems, e.g. systemic conditions such as renal failure, severe pain, drugs, etc.

Q3.11 Is vomiting always associated with nausea?

A: No, vomiting in patients with increased intracranial pressure may be explosive and not preceded by nausea.

Q3.12 Having asked about frequency of vomiting, what should be asked about vomitus?

A: • Amount.
    • Colour.[1]
    • Content.[2]

    1. Special attention should be paid to presence of blood in vomitus (haematemesis). If patient bleeds profusely vomitus may consist of dark, bright-red blood. Often, however, vomitus has blackish appearance with sediment of 'coffee grounds'.
    2. In patients with a pharyngo-oesophageal pouch, lower oesophageal obstruction or pyloric stenosis, recognizable food may be vomited a long time after it was eaten. Faecal vomiting indicates a gastrocolic fistula or low intestinal obstruction.

CHANGE OF BOWEL HABIT

Q3.13 Why should patients complaining of a change in bowel function[1] be examined carefully?

A: A change in bowel habit may indicate the presence of serious pathology such as carcinoma of the rectum or large bowel.

1. Enquire carefully about normal bowel function. 'Normal' bowel function may vary from several motions daily to once every 3 or 4 days.

Q3.14 What is tenesmus?

A: Tenesmus is a feeling of incomplete emptying of the bowel. It is often associated with inflammatory disease of the bowel and rectal carcinoma.

DIARRHOEA

Q3.15 What points should be noted about diarrhoea?

A: • Frequency.
   • Amount.
   • Semiformed or liquid.
   • Colour.[1]
   • Association with abdominal pain or rectal pain.
   • Association with incontinence.[2]
   • Associated with fever.
   • Use of purgatives.
   • Contacts.[3]

1. Stools pale, bulky and smelly in steatorrhoea, pale in obstructive jaundice, black from iron ingestion or following gastrointestinal bleeding, watery in severe cholera.
2. May point to a neurological problem.
3. Important in epidemics of food poisoning, cholera, etc.

BLOODY DIARRHOEA AND BLOOD IN STOOL

Q3.16 What are the most frequent causes of bloody diarrhoea?

A: • Carcinoma of colon.
   • Ulcerative colitis.
   • Shigella infections.
   • Amoebic dysentery.

Q3.17 What are the most common causes of bleeding from the rectum and streaking of the stool with blood?

A: • Haemorrhoids (piles).[1]
   • Carcinoma of colon and rectum.

   1. Remember that haemorrhoids may be a sign of portal hypertension.

Q3.18 Is abdominal distension always an important sign of alimentary disease?

A: In developed countries no, because of the high frequency of obesity, but in developing countries abdominal distension is commonly a symptom which should be taken seriously, especially if it occurs in individuals who are thin or losing weight.

Q3.19 What, apart from pregnancy and obesity, may abdominal distension indicate?

A: • Accumulation of fluid in abdomen (ascites).
   • Gaseous distension as a result of intestinal obstruction or paralytic ileus.
   • Splenic and hepatic enlargement or other masses.[1]

   1. Other masses include ovarian cysts, polycystic kidneys and, in certain developing countries, hydatid cysts.

SYMPTOMS OF LIVER DISEASE

Q3.20 What are the common symptoms of acute liver disease such as viral hepatitis?

A: • General malaise.[1]

- Anorexia.
- Nausea and vomiting.
- Fever.
- Distaste for cigarettes.
- Jaundice.

1. Symptoms of general malaise may precede onset of jaundice by up to 2 weeks.

Q3.21 What are the common symptoms of chronic liver disease?

A:
- Swelling of abdomen and ankles due to oedema.
- Haematemesis and melaena.
- Pruritus.
- Loss of libido.
- Amenorrhoea.
- Personality changes – confusion and drowsiness.[1]

1. Such changes point to the likelihood of portosystemic encephalopathy.

JAUNDICE

Q3.22 What questions should be asked of the jaundiced patient?[1]

A:
- Duration of jaundice.
- Whether fluctuating or progressive.
- Colour of urine and stool.
- Anorexia and nausea.
- Associated pain and weight loss.
- Itch.
- Fever or rigors.
- Distaste for smoking.
- Alcohol intake.
- Recent history of blood transfusion and injections including traditional treatments on skin.
- Drug history including drug addiction.
- Sickle-cell disease and other blood diseases.
- Other family members or friends with jaundice.
- Homosexuality.
- Travel abroad.

1. Questions should be asked which are appropriate to the patient's circumstances.

EXAMINATION

GENERAL EXAMINATION

Q3.23 Physical examination will often reveal evidence of alimentary disease or liver disease in other parts of the body. Name these parts

A: • Hands.
   • Face.
   • Eyes.
   • Mouth.
   • Skin.

Q3.24 What signs should be looked for on examination of the hands?

A: • Leukonychia (pallor of nails).[1]
   • Finger clubbing.[2]
   • Palmar erythema.[3]
   • Dupuytren's contracture.[4]
   • Asterixis (flapping tremor).

1. Leukonychia may be due to anaemia or hypo-albuminaemia.
2. Finger clubbing may be found in hepatic cirrhosis, ulcerative colitis, Crohn's disease, and coeliac disease.
3. A sign of chronic liver disease, but also seen in pregnancy, thyrotoxicosis and rheumatoid arthritis.
4. Seen in alcoholic cirrhosis.

Q3.25 What signs may be present in the face?

A: • Cachectic appearance.
   • Parotid swelling.[1]

1. May be seen in malnourished patients and alcoholics.

Q3.26 What signs may be present in the eyes?

A: • Jaundice.
• Pallor of conjunctivae.

Q3.27 What signs should be looked for in the mouth?

A: • Furring of tongue.[1]
• Atrophic glossitis.[2]
• Mouth ulcers.[3]
• Angular stomatitis.
• Candidiasis.
• Jaundice.[4]
• Telangiectasia.[5]
• Spots of pigmentation around the mouth.[6]

1. Marked furring may be seen in febrile patients, in uraemia and liver failure.
2. Evidence of iron, vitamin B_{12}, folic acid, riboflavin and nicotinic acid deficiency. It may also be a manifestation of coeliac disease.
3. These may be associated with inflammatory bowel disease, e.g. Crohn's disease.
4. Yellow coloration may first appear in the frenulum of the tongue in jaundiced patients.
5. Hereditary haemorrhagic telangiectasia.
6. May point to Peutz–Jeghers syndrome, i.e. presence of small bowel polyposis.

Q3.28 What should be looked for on examination of the skin?

A: • Jaundice.
• Scratch marks.[1]
• Pigmentation.[2]
• Bruises.[3]
• Therapeutic marks or evidence of intravenous drug abuse.[4]
• Spider naevi.[5]
• Dermatitis.[6]
• Gynaecomastia.[7]
• Xanthomas.[8]

1. Result of the pruritus associated with cholestasis.
2. May be increased in haemochromatosis.
3. May indicate bleeding tendency in patients with liver disease.
4. May be associated with viral hepatitis.
5. Found mostly in anterior upper chest, neck and face. May be difficult to see in dark skin.
6. May be associated with vitamin deficiency, e.g. pellagra.
7. Associated with liver cirrhosis and spironolactone therapy for ascites.
8. Seen in primary biliary cirrhosis.

EXAMINATION OF ABDOMEN

INSPECTION

Q3.29 What should be looked for on inspection as you sit or kneel at patient's bedside?

A: • Shape – scaphoid or distended.
   • Skin lesions – surgical scars, therapeutic marks, striae.
   • Umbilicus.
   • Veins.[1]
   • Visible pulsations.[2]
   • Visible peristalsis.[3]
   • Abdominal wall movement.[4]
   • Hernial orifices.[5]
   • Genitalia.[6]

1. Dilated veins may occur in portal hypertension and inferior vena caval obstruction.
2. Visible aortic pulsations may be normal in thin individuals. A pulsating liver may be seen in tricuspid regurgitation.
3. An important sign of intestinal obstruction.
4. Diminished or absent movement of the abdominal wall muscles is seen in peritonitis.
5. Look for hernia and lymphadenopathy.
6. Do not forget to examine perianal area for evidence of haemorrhoids, fistulae, fissures, etc.

Q3.30 Ascites is a frequent cause of abdominal distension. What are common causes of ascites?

A:
- Portal hypertension.
- Intra-abdominal malignancy.
- Congestive cardiac failure including constrictive pericarditis.
- Nephrotic syndrome.
- Tuberculosis.
- Peritonitis.
- Abdominal trauma.

Q3.31 In which of these conditions will ascites be an exudate?

A:
- Tuberculosis.
- Intra-abdominal malignancy.
- Peritonitis.

Q3.32 How do you distinguish an exudate from a transudate?

A: In a exudate the protein content will be > 30 g/l whilst in a transudate the protein concentration will be < 30 g/l. The cell count will also often be increased in an exudate.

Q3.33 What else may cause diffuse abdominal distension apart from ascites (fluid)?

A:
- Obesity (fat).
- Gas (flatus).
- Pregnancy (fetus).
- Massive splenomegaly.
- Ovarian and hydatid cysts.

PALPATION

Q3.34 What important signs of peritonitis are elicited on palpation?

A:
- Guarding (involuntary muscle contraction).[1]
- Rigidity.[2]
- Rebound tenderness.

1. Indicates localized peritonitis.
2. Indicates diffuse peritonitis, but distinguish from voluntary contraction of abdominal muscles in anxious patients.

Q3.35 What points should be noted about abdominal masses?

A:
- Site.
- Size.
- Shape or contour.
- Tenderness.
- Consistency.
- Mobility.
- Fluctuation.

Palpation of the Liver

Q3.36 Is the liver sometimes palpable in normal subjects?

A: Yes, It may be palpable on deep inspiration in the epigastrium and just below the right costal margin. It may also be pushed downwards in patients with emphysema.

Q3.37 What is Reidel's lobe?

A: An anatomical variant of the right lobe of liver, which may be confused with hepatomegaly or an enlarged right kidney.

Q3.38 The causes of hepatomegaly are many. When faced with the differential diagnosis of hepatomegaly it is best to think of disease groups. **Which disease groups include most of the common causes of hepatomegaly?**

A:
- Parasitic and infectious causes.[1]
- Cirrhosis of the liver.
- Malignancy, especially hepatocellular carcinoma (hepatoma).
- Congestive disorders.[2]
- Diseases of the blood and reticuloendothelial system.
- Miscellaneous.[3]

1. The most common causes of hepatomegaly in the developing world – causes to be considered in this group include malaria, viral hepatitis, tuberculosis, schistosomiasis, pyogenic and amoebic abscesses.
2. These include congestive cardiac failure, constrictive pericarditis, tricuspid regurgitation, occlusion of hepatic vein (Budd–Chiari syndrome).
3. These include infiltrative disorders, such as amyloidosis, and fatty liver.

Q3.39 What points should be noted about an enlarged liver?

A: • Consistency – firm or soft.
   • Regularity or smoothness of its surface and edge.
   • Tenderness.
   • Degree of enlargement in centimetres.
   • Presence of pulsation.[1]
   • Presence of bruits.[2]

1. Pulsations may be seen in tricuspid regurgitation.
2. A bruit may be heard over a hepatocellular carcinoma.

Q3.40 What signs may be found in chronic liver disease?

A: • Jaundice.
   • Skin changes.[1]
   • Hepatomegaly.[2]
   • Splenomegaly.[3]
   • Ascites and oedema.
   • Dilated veins on abdomen.
   • Endocrine charges.[4]
   • Parotid enlargement.
   • Portosystemic encephalopathy.[5]

1. These include spider naevi above the nipple line, darkening of skin in haemochromatosis, palmar erythema, Dupuytren's contracture and, rarely, clubbing. Xanthomas may be seen in primary biliary cirrhosis. There may be loss of body hair.

2. The liver is not usually palpable in well-established cirrhosis.
3. Splenomegaly may be an important sign of portal hypertension.
4. These include gynaecomastia and testicular atrophy.
5. Signs of encephalopathy include drowsiness, reversal of the normal sleep rhythm, convulsions, coma and flapping tremor. Test for evidence of constructional apraxia by asking the patient to draw a star and intellectual function by the serial sevens test.

Q3.41 What complications may be associated with cirrhosis of the liver?

A: • Portal hypertension and gastrointestinal haemorrhage.
   • Ascites.
   • Portosystemic encephalopathy.
   • Renal failure.
   • Primary liver cell cancer (hepatoma).

Palpation of Other Organs

Q3.42 Is the spleen ever felt in normal subjects?

A: No, before it can be felt it must be enlarged by two to three times.

Q3.43 What are the five characteristics which help to distinguish splenomegaly from enlargement of the kidney?

A: 1. It moves downwards on respiration.
   2. The fingers of the examiner's hand cannot be pushed under the left costal margin to get above the mass.
   3. A notch may be felt on the medial border.
   4. There is dullness on percussion over the mass. (The left kidney is crossed by a band of resonance due to the overlying colon.)
   5. It may be possible to insert fingers in the space between its posterior edge and the spinal muscles posteriorly.

Q3.44 As with hepatomegaly the causes of splenomegaly are many. Think of causes within broad disease groups. **Which disease groups include most of the common and not-so-common causes of splenomegaly?**

A:
- Parasitic and infectious diseases.[1]
- Diseases of the blood and reticuloendothelial system.[2]
- Congestive disorders.[3]
- Miscellaneous causes.[4]

1. These are numerous and include malaria (tropical splenomegaly syndrome), viral hepatitis, typhoid, bacterial endocarditis, visceral leishmaniasis (kala-azar), brucellosis and infectious mononucleosis.
2. These include haemolytic diseases, haemoglobinopathies and leukaemias.
3. Hepatic cirrhosis and portal hypertension is the most common cause in this group. Splenic or portal vein thromboses are other less common causes.
4. These include rheumatoid arthritis (Felty's syndrome) and infiltrative disorders, such as amyloidosis and Gaucher's disease. Other rare causes include cysts, abscess and metastases.

Q3.45 What are the major causes of massive splenomegaly?

A:
- Tropical splenomegaly syndrome (TSS).
- Visceral leishmaniasis (kala-azar).
- Chronic myeloid leukaemia.
- Myelofibrosis.

Q3.46 Sometimes it may be difficult to distinguish between a large spleen and a large left kidney. **What features will help in the identification of the kidney?**

A:
- The kidney moves downwards on inspiration but to a lesser extent then the spleen.
- The examiner's fingers can usually get above it.
- It may cause bulging of the flank.
- It is bimanually palpable.
- There will be resonance on percussion if overlaid by the colon.

Q3.47 What other masses may sometimes be difficult to distinguish from a large spleen or large left kidney?

A: • Enlarged left lobe of liver.
   • Tumour arising from the stomach.
   • Pancreatic tumour or cyst.
   • Tumour or large amount of hard faeces in the colon.
   • Tumour or cyst of ovary.
   • Tumour arising from the left adrenal gland.

Q3.48 What else should be examined under the heading of palpation?

A: • Uterus and bladder.
   • Other masses.
   • Palpation for fluid thrill.
   • Ballottment/dipping.
   • Succussion splash.[1]
   • Hernial orifices[2] and groins for lymphadenopathy and infective skin lesions.
   • Anorectal examination.[3]
   • Genitalia.

1. Identified by rocking patient from side to side. Only abnormal if still present 2–3 hours after a meal.
2. As well as inguinal and femoral hernias, note also presence of umbilical, epigastric and incisional hernias.
3. In males palpate prostate, and in females cervix and lateral fornices. In all the anal canal should be carefully examined for evidence of inflammation, ulceration, fissures, fistulae-in-ano, abscesses, skin tags, warts and haemorrhoids.

Q3.49 How do you distinguish between an indirect and direct inguinal hernia?

A: • By observing the direction of the expansile impulse induced by asking the patient to cough. An indirect hernia passes through the internal inguinal ring, and then, if large enough, passes obliquely through the inguinal canal and through the external inguinal ring into the scrotum. The expansile impulse will therefore follow this route. A direct inguinal hernia, however, protrudes directly forwards through the posterior wall of the inguinal canal medial to the internal ring and, only very rarely, pushes its way through the external inguinal ring into the scrotum. The expansile impulse therefore is generally directly forwards.

- If an indirect hernia is reducible it can be controlled by placing a fingertip over the internal inguinal ring, about 1/2 inch (12 mm) above the femoral pulse which can be palpated at the mid-inguinal point. A direct inguinal hernia will not be controlled by pressure over the internal ring.

Q3.50 How may you distinguish between an indirect inguinal hernia and a femoral hernia?

A: An indirect inguinal hernia which protrudes through the external inguinal ring can be palpated above and medial to the pubic tubercle, whilst a femoral hernia lies below and lateral to this bony landmark.

PERCUSSION

Q3.51 What uses are made of percussion in the examination of the abdomen?

A: • To confirm upper and lower borders of the liver.
- To elicit shifting dullness in patients with ascites.
- Identification of enlarged bladder (dull to percussion).

AUSCULTATION

Q3.52 What sounds should be listened for on auscultation of the abdomen?

A: • Bowel sounds.[1]
- Vascular bruits.[2]
- Hepatic bruit.[3]
- Splenic rubs.[4]

1. Bowel sounds will be increased in intensity and frequency in conditions of increased intestinal motility, e.g. in diarrhoea. In early intestinal obstruction they

are also increased and may have a high-pitched, metallic, tinkling quality. In peritonitis bowel sounds are absent.

2. For example, renal artery stenosis.
3. May be heard over hepatocellular carcinoma or hepatic metastases.
4. May be heard over area of splenic infarction.

PLAN FOR EXAMINATION OF THE ALIMENTARY SYSTEM

General	Hands, eyes, mouth, skin.
Inspection	Shape (contour)
	Movement of abdominal wall
	Umbilicus
	Veins
	Visible pulsations
	Visible peristalsis
Palpation	Tenderness, guarding, rigidity
	Liver
	Spleen
	Kidney
	Masses
	Fluid thrill
Percussion	Shifting dullness
	Upper and lower borders of the liver
Auscultation	Bowel sounds
	Bruits
Examination of groins and genitalia	
Rectal examination	

4
THE KIDNEY AND URINARY TRACT

SYMPTOMS OF DISEASES OF THE KIDNEY AND URINARY TRACT

Q4.1 What are the principal symptoms of renal disease and diseases of the urinary tract? (Remember that extensive renal disease may exist without symptoms)

A:
- Abdominal pain including pain in loins, lumbosacral region and genitalia.
- Dysuria (burning pain on passing urine).[1]
- Frequency of micturition.[1]
- Urgency.[1]
- Nocturia.[2]
- Incontinence.[3]
- Retention of urine.[4]
- Hesitancy, poor urinary stream and terminal dribbling.[5]
- Oliguria, anuria.
- Polyuria.[6]
- Haematuria.[7]
- Chyluria.[8]
- Pneumaturia.[9]
- Urethral discharge.
- Enuresis.[10]

1. Common symptoms indicating irritation of bladder and urethra by infection, stones or tumour. Frequency refers to the frequent passage of small volumes of urine. Urgency and precipitancy are also common symptoms in diseases of the nervous system such as multiple sclerosis.

2. Nocturia, i.e. the need to pass urine during the night is a common habit and may therefore be normal. It is, however, often an early symptom of chronic renal failure. It may also be a symptom of heart failure.
3. May be due to cystocele (stress incontinence) or disease of the nervous system.
4. May be due to mechanical obstruction or neurological disease.
5. Common symptoms of prostatic hypertrophy.
6. Refers to the frequent passage of large volumes of urine, e.g. in diabetes and chronic renal failure.
7. Haematuria may occur in cystitis. If haematuria is associated with colic it is probably due to renal stones. If terminal it suggests schistosomiasis in countries where this disease occurs. Other causes include glomerulonephritis, carcinoma and renal papillary necrosis.
8. Seen in filariasis.
9. Seen in vesicocolic fistula.
10. A common problem, which may be seen in adults as well as children.

Q4.2 How may glomerulonephritis present?

A: • Asymptomatic proteinuria and/or microscopic haematuria.
• Acute nephritic syndrome.
• Nephrotic syndrome.
• Chronic renal failure.

Q4.3 In patients with renal failure (acute or chronic) the history should seek to identify possible prerenal, renal and postrenal causes. **If the cause is not immediately obvious, e.g. haemorrhage or burns, what symptoms, and relevant information in the past medical and social history, should be looked for with care?**

A: • Vomiting and diarrhoea.[1]
• Jaundice.[2]
• Recent sore throat, otitis media or cellulitis.[3]
• Drug intake.[4]

- Occupation.[5]
- Family history of renal disease.[6]
- Residence in warm climates.[7]
- Recent abdominal or pelvic surgery.
- History of prostatism.
- History of diabetes, hypertension, chronic pyelone-phritis, systemic lupus erythematosus, gout, multiple myeloma, schistosomiasis.

1. May result in severe volume depletion, e.g. cholera.
2. Renal failure may occur in association with liver failure (hepatorenal syndrome).
3. Streptococcal infection of throat may precede onset of the acute nephritic syndrome by 1–3 weeks.
4. A wide variety of drugs are potentially nephrotoxic.
5. May result from exposure to chemicals.
6. For example, polycystic renal disease.
7. May be relevant in patients with renal stones.

Q4.4 Chronic renal failure may involve almost every body system. **What symptoms may be seen in chronic renal failure attributable to involvement of the cardio-vascular system and to disturbances in water and electrolyte balance?**

A: • Breathlessness.[1]
   • Postural fainting.[2]
   • Lethargy and weakness.[3]
   • Chest pain.[4]
   • Palpitations.[5]

1. May be due to salt and water overload, acidosis (Kussmaul's respiration) and heart failure.
2. Due to salt and water depletion.
3. Due to salt and water depletion or hypokalaemia.
4. May be due to angina resulting from anaemia or due to pericarditis.
5. May result from arrhythmias due to hyperkalaemia.

Q4.5 What symptoms may result from involvement of the gastrointestinal tract?

A: • Anaemia.
  • Nausea.
  • Vomiting.
  • Hiccough.
  • Diarrhoea.
  • Haematemesis and melaena.

Q4.6 What symptoms may result from involvement of the haemopoietic system?

A: • Breathlessness.[1]
  • Tiredness.[1]
  • Headache.[1]
  • Excessive bruising and bleeding.[2]

  1. Symptoms of anaemia.
  2. The result of platelet abnormalities.

Q4.7 What symptoms may result from involvement of the respiratory system?

A: • Breathlessness.
  • Haemoptysis.
  • Pleuritic chest pain.

Q4.8 What symptoms may result from involvement of the musculoskeletal system?

A: • Weakness.[1]
  • Bone pain.[1]

  1. Symptoms resulting from renal osteodystrophy.

Q4.9 What symptoms may result from involvement of the nervous system and eyes?

A: • Depression.
  • Headache.
  • Drowsiness.
  • Symptoms of peripheral neuropathy.

- Visual loss.[1]
- Seizures.
- Coma.

1. Due to hypertensive retinopathy or retinal vascular thrombosis.

Q4.10 Can the kidneys be palpated in normal subjects?

A: Usually no, but the lower border of the right kidney may be felt in thin patients.

Q4.11 What signs may be observed on inspection in a patient with chronic renal failure?

A: • Skin changes.[1]
   • Pallor of mucosa.
   • Oedema including facial puffiness.
   • Leukonychia.[2]
   • Ulcers on the lips, evidence of fungal infection in the mouth.[3]
   • Difficulties in walking, rising from a chair, etc.[4]
   • Growth retardation in children and delayed puberty.
   • Uraemic flap.

1. Skin may be dry and itchy and have a dirty yellow-brown appearance. There may be bruises and scratch marks and, in terminal uraemia, 'uraemic frost' on the forehead.
2. White nails due to hypoalbuminaemia.
3. These may occur in patients on immunosuppressive drugs.
4. May be due to renal osteodystrophy or peripheral neuropathy.

5

THE REPRODUCTIVE SYSTEM AND SEXUALLY TRANSMITTED DISEASES

SYMPTOMS RELATED TO DIMINISHED OR DISORDERED FUNCTION OF THE GENITALIA AND SEXUALLY TRANSMITTED DISEASES

Q5.1 What symptoms reflect failure, or disordered function, of the ovaries and the reproductive system in females?

A:
- Primary amenorrhoea.[1]
- Secondary amenorrhoea.[2]
- Other menstrual disorders.[3]
- Loss of libido.[4]
- Subfertility.[5]
- Reduction in breast size.
- Galactorrhoea.[6]
- Dyspareunia.[7]
- Loss of body hair.
- Short stature.
- Delayed puberty.[8]
- Precocious puberty.[9]
- Hirsuties.[10]

1. Failure to start menstruation by the age of 16 years.
2. Loss of periods for 3 months in a woman who has previously been menstruating.
3. Enquire about regularity and duration of periods, amount of blood loss and whether painful (dysmenorrhoea).
4. Loss of sexual desire. May be due to tiredness,

anxiety, depression, physical illness, as well as loss of ovarian function.

5. Defined as failure to conceive after one year of unprotected intercourse.

6. Galactorrhoea may be spontaneous or occur on expression.

7. Painful sexual intercourse may result from loss of vaginal lubrication as a result of oestrogen deficiency (see Q5.3).

8. Puberty is said to be delayed if there are no signs of pubertal development by age 15 or 16.

9. Puberty is considered precocious if menarche and secondary sexual characteristics occur before the age of 9 in girls and boys.

10. On examination look for evidence of virilization (cliteromegaly, male distribution of body hair, acne).

Q5.2 What symptoms may result from failure, or disordered function, of the genitalia and reproductive system in males?

A: • Loss of libido.
• Impotence.[1]
• Subfertility.
• Gynaecomastia.[2]
• Short stature.
• Delayed puberty.
• Loss of body hair.
• Precocious puberty.
• Hirsuties.

1. Defined as inability to achieve or sustain an erection for satisfactory sexual intercourse. There are many causes, both psychological and physical. Enquire about drug history, alcohol intake, anxieties and diabetes. Organic impotence is suggested by failure to experience nocturnal erections and emissions, and absence of erection when bladder is full. If due to hypogonadism testes are small and soft, and there may loss of body hair.

2. Occurs in up to 50% of normal boys at puberty.

SYMPTOMS OF SEXUALLY TRANSMITTED DISEASE

Q5.3 About what symptoms should you ask a man or a woman who may have a sexually transmitted disease?

A:

Men	Women	Symptoms common to both sexes
• Urethral discharge[1] • Dysuria • Frequency • Balanitis • Painful or swollen scrotum[2] • Anorectal symptoms[3]	• Vaginal discharge[1,4] • Dyspareunia[5] • Low abdominal pain • Vulvitis	• Genital ulceration[6] • Pubic and genital itch[7] • Genital rash

1. Enquire about duration, colour and amount; gonorrhoea, for example, is associated with a purulent discharge.
2. Such a symptom may also point to other conditions such as malignancy and torsion of the testes.
3. These include pain, itch, rectal discharge, tenesmus, constipation and diarrhoea.
4. Enquire if it has an offensive smell, or is associated with itch. Itch, for example, may be due to candidal infection.
5. Dyspareunia may be due to a wide variety of causes, both physical and psychological.
6. Ask if lesion is painful. Painful ulcers, for example, occur in herpes and chancroid, whilst in lymphogranuloma venereum ulcers are painless. Enquire also if ulcers are recurrent.
7. May be related to pediculosis pubis or scabies.

Q5.4 What additional points should be noted in the past medical and social history of a person whom you consider may have a sexually transmitted disease?

A: • Past history of genitourinary problems.
 • Past history of jaundice (viral hepatitis).
 • Obstetric history.[1]
 • Menstrual history.[2]

- Recent abortion.
- Condom and contraceptive use.
- Drug history.[3]
- Residence in the Tropics.[4]
- Sexual orientation.[5]
- Sexual contacts.[6]
- History of prostitution.

1. Enquire about previous ectopic pregnancies, stillbirths, abortions, babies with ophthalmia neonatorum.
2. Pelvic inflammatory disease may lead to change in the menstrual cycle, but remember possibility of ectopic pregnancy in someone with a missed period and unilateral lower abdominal pain.
3. Is there a history of drug abuse? Has the patient taken antibiotics in the recent past?
4. For example, patient may have chancroid, lympho-granuloma venereum, granuloma inguinale or HIV infection.
5. Patients may understandably be very reluctant to reveal their sexual orientation, and much experience and sensitivity is required in this area of history-taking.
6. Were contacts regular or casual? What was specific nature of sexual activity? Is patient engaged in high-risk behaviour? How long has it been between onset of symptoms and risk of infection?

COMMENT: TAKING A HISTORY AND HIV INFECTION

Taking a history from a persons who may be at risk of infection with the human immunodeficiency virus may be difficult and embarrassing for both patient and doctor. Specific questions should be asked sensitively as follows, and only after you have established a good rapport with the patient. Questions asked should be relevant to the culture, circumstances, town, country, etc. in which the patient lives.

For men:
- Have you ever had sex with a man?
- Have you ever had sex with a woman who used intravenous drugs?
- Have you ever had sex with a prostitute (male or female)?

For women:
- Have you ever had sex with a man who you know or suspect is bisexual (or who has had sex with other men)?
- Have you ever had sex with a man who used intravenous drugs?

For both sexes:
- Have you ever used intravenous drugs?
- Have you ever had a blood transfusion?
- How many sexual partners would you estimate you have had in the last 3–6 months?
- Have you ever had sex with someone who subsequently developed AIDS?
- Have you ever paid money or received money for sex?

EXAMINATION OF MALE GENITALIA AND OF PATIENTS WITH SEXUALLY TRANSMITTED DISEASE

Q5.5 Inspection and palpation of males and females who may have a sexually transmitted disease should be carried out in a systematic way. **In what order should you proceed?**

A: 1. Males – Inspect in a good light:
- Examine the lower abdominal skin, perineum and upper inner thighs for rashes, spots, lice, inflammation and warts.
- Examine the scrotal skin including the posterior aspect for rashes, ulcers, etc., and palpate the testes, epididymes and spermatic cords for swellings and tenderness.
- Examine the penile skin and, if present, retract the prepuce, inspecting the coronal sulcus, glans penis and urethral meatus for rashes, spots, warts, sores, inflammation and urethral discharge.
- Examine the perineal skin and anus from the rear, for spots, rashes, warts and anal discharge.

2. Females:
  - Examine the lower abdominal skin, perineum and upper inner thighs for rashes, spots, lice, inflammation and warts.
  - Examine the labia majora and labia minora for sores, rashes, spots, inflammation, discharges and warts.
  - Examine the introitus (vulva) for swelling of ducts of Bartholin's glands and inflammation, the urethral meatus and lower vagina for discharges, rashes, spots, sores and warts.[1]
  - Examine the perineal skin and anus from the rear, for spots, rashes, warts and anal discharge.

  1. An upper vaginal and cervical examination should be carried out when indicated.

Q5.6 Sexually transmitted diseases may be associated with involvement of other parts of the body apart from the genitalia. **What parts should be carefully examined?**

A:
  - Skin.[1]
  - Mouth.[2]
  - Anus and rectum.
  - Eyes.[3]
  - Joints.[4]
  - Sites of possible lymph node enlargement.
  - Central nervous system.[5]

1. Look for evidence of skin rashes, opportunistic infection, Kaposi's sarcoma, chancres, ulcers, gummata, etc.
2. Look for evidence of opportunistic infections, gummata, leukoplakia, Kaposi's sarcoma, chancres, etc.
3. Conjunctivitis may be caused by the herpes virus, gonococcus or chlamydia. Conjunctivitis and iritis may also be associated with Reiter's disease.
4. Joints may be involved in disseminated gonococcal infection, Reiter's disease and HIV infection, Charcot's joints in tabes dorsalis are rarely seen nowadays.
5. The nervous system is commonly involved in HIV infection and, rarely nowadays, in syphilis.

6
THE NERVOUS SYSTEM

THE NERVOUS SYSTEM AND EYES

Q6.1 What conditions are necessary for the successful examination of the nervous system?

A: • A basic knowledge of anatomy.
   • The necessary skills for examination.
   • Ability to relate well to the patient since the patient's cooperation is essential.
   • The necessary tools.
   • A positive attitude.

Q6.2 The correct interpretation of signs in diseases of the nervous system depends greatly on the examiner's knowledge of basic anatomy. **Are you familiar with the anatomy of the following parts of the nervous system?**

A: • The cerebrum (major features).
   • The internal capsule.
   • The motor pathways.
   • The sensory pathways.
   • The main features which would be seen in cross-sectional views of the mid-brain, pons, medulla and spinal cord.
   • The cerebellum.
   • The anatomy of visual field defects and eye movements.
   • The origin and course of the other cranial nerves.
   • The blood supply to the brain and the circle of Willis.
   • The major peripheral nerves and muscle groups.
   • The dermatomes (cutaneous areas supplied by sensory roots).

Q6.3 What tools are necessary for adequate examination?

A: • A tendon hammer, preferably with a long flexible handle and round rubber head.
   • A tuning fork to test vibration sense (low frequency, 128 Hz).
   • Disposable Sterolets or needles for testing pain sensation.
   • Cotton wool to test touch.
   • Some means of testing temperature sensation.[1]
   • An ophthalmoscope.

   1. Often not tested during routine examination but important when testing sensory loss in patients with leprosy.

Q6.4 In the diagnosis of neurological disease the history is of crucial importance. Start from the beginning of the patient's story and follow its progression step by step. When you put the story together you should have a clear picture of the natural history of the disease, and therefore important clues to the underlying nature of the disease process. To ensure that all important symptoms have been covered in your patient's history what would your check list of neurological symptoms be?

A: • Mental state including memory,[1] hallucinations[2] and delusions,[3] and mood.
   • Insomnia.[4]
   • Loss of consciousness.[5]
   • Headache.[6]
   • Visual disturbance.[7]
   • Giddiness, vertigo.[8]
   • Dizziness.[9]
   • Tinnitus.[10]
   • Deafness.[11]
   • Aural pain or discharge.
   • Dysphagia.[12]
   • Weakness or paralysis of limbs.
   • Tremor.[13]

- Numbness, paraesthesia (pins and needles).[14]
- Loss of sensation.[15]
- Bladder and bowel function.[16]

1. Memory is often subdivided into long-/medium-term memory and short-term memory. It may be important to speak to relatives or friends about changes in the patient's mental state.
2. Subjectively realistic perception of objects, sounds, and smells and tastes that have no reality.
3. False beliefs regarding the self or people or objects outside the self that persist despite evidence to the contrary.
4. May be an important symptom of depression or the result of pain or cough.
5. Ask about onset, sudden or slow, whether preceded by warning, of tongue-biting or incontinence, duration, after-effects, precipitating cause(s).
6. Character, site, duration, association with other symptoms, e.g. vomiting.
7. Seeing double (diplopia), loss of visual acuity, field defect.
8. Feeling of loss of balance with the impression that the surroundings are whirling around.
9. A symptom whose significance is often difficult to interpret. In contrast to vertigo, dizziness refers to a subjective feeling of unsteadiness.
10. A subjective awareness of noise, often a hissing sound, in the absence of any external stimuli.
11. Ask about onset, whether sudden or slow; is deafness progressive, constant or fluctuant; are one or both ears affected?
12. May be associated with bulbar or pseudobulbar palsies.
13. See Q6.118.
14. May be an important symptom of peripheral neuropathy.
15. Very important in leprosy and is the cause of injuries to hands and feet.
16. Frequency and incontinence are associated with

bilateral upper motor neurone lesions. Incontinence also often follows a unilateral cerebrovascular accident but usually recovers within weeks or months. Dementia is also associated with incontinence.

PAST MEDICAL HISTORY

Q6.5 What problems may be of importance in the past medical history of patients with neurological diseases? (Attention should be paid only to those problems which are of relevance to the particular neurological problem with which you are faced)

A:
- Trauma.[1]
- Cardiovascular diseases, especially hypertension and rheumatic heart disease.
- Respiratory diseases such as pneumonia.[2]
- Haematological diseases such as bleeding disorders.
- Hepatocellular failure.[3]
- Renal failure.[4]
- Joint and connective tissue diseases.[5]
- Endocrine and metabolic diseases, especially diabetes.[6]
- Neoplastic disease.[7]
- Sexually transmitted disease.[8]
- Tuberculosis and leprosy.
- Recent viral infection.[9]

1. Of the utmost importance in patients with suspected subdural and extradural haemorrhage. Remember that the latent period in chronic subdural haematoma between injury and onset of symptoms may vary from weeks to months. Head injury may also be associated with infectious diseases such as pneumococcal meningitis and tetanus.
2. Confusional states may result from hypoxia, especially in the elderly.
3. See Q3.21, 3.40.
4. See Q4.9.
5. See Q8.9.

6. Hypoglycaemia, hypocalcaemia and hyponatraemia may be associated with seizures. Hypothyroidism may be associated with the carpal tunnel syndrome, cerebellar disease and dementia. Think of neurological problems associated with other endocrine and metabolic diseases.
7. There is a wide variety of non-metastatic neurological manifestations of malignancy.
8. Syphilis and HIV infection are associated with a wide variety of neurological disorders.
9. May precede post-infective polyneuropathy (Guillain–Barré syndrome).

SOCIAL/FAMILY/DRUG HISTORY

Q6.6 What points should be noted in the social, family and drug history of someone with a neurological problem?

A: • Smoking.[1]
   • Alcohol.
   • Drug history.[2]
   • Dietary history.[3]
   • Occupation.[4]
   • Sexual history.
   • Travel abroad.[5]
   • Contact with tuberculosis, meningitis and polio.
   • Family history of neurological disease.[6]

1. A risk factor for cerebrovascular disease.
2. Phenothiazines, for example, may be associated with parkinsonism, metoclopramide with severe dystonic reactions, isoniazid with peripheral neuropathy. Many drugs can cause a wide variety of neurological disorders.
3. A poor diet may be associated with deficiency of thiamine, nicotinic acid, pyridoxine and folic acid.
4. Occupation may involve exposure to toxic substances such as lead.
5. Important if patient has suspected cerebral malaria, poliomyelitis, etc.

6. For example, neurofibromatosis, Huntington's disease, Freidreich's' ataxia, etc.

EXAMINATION: HIGHER CEREBRAL FUNCTION

LEVEL OF CONSCIOUSNESS

Q6.7 In patients with an altered level of consciousness how may their clinical state be described?

A: By use of the following clinical grading:
- fully conscious,
- drowsiness,
- delirium,[1]
- stupor,[2]
- coma.[3]

By use of the Glasgow Coma Scale.

1. Delirium is an acute confusional state marked by clouding of consciousness, decreased alertness, irritability, agitation, sensory misinterpretation and often hallucinations.
2. A state of marked unresponsiveness but arousal possible by stimulation.
3. A state of 'unarousable unresponsiveness' or, in the Glasgow Coma Scale, 'not obeying commands, no words uttered and eyes never opened'.

MOOD OR AFFECT

Q6.8 What is meant by the patient's mood or affect?

A: Whether elated or depressed, agitated or anxious.

BEHAVIOUR AND APPEARANCE

Q6.9 If patient has a very unkempt appearance what might this suggest?

A: Possibility of alcoholism, drug addiction or of some psychotic illness.

MEMORY AND INTELLIGENCE

Q6.10 Memory is often classified into short-term and medium/long-term memory. **How may you assess short-term and medium/long-term memory?**

A: • Short-term memory: the patient is asked to recall a test name and address after 2 and 5 minutes.
   • Medium/long-term memory: the patient is asked about well-known aspects of current affairs, e.g. name of the President, Prime Minister, etc. (Questions to assess memory and intelligence must be appropriate to the patient's culture and circumstances.)

SPEECH

Q6.11 If you have a patient who appears unable to speak or who speaks with difficulty what conditions should you consider?

A: • Dysphasia.[1]
   • Dysarthria.
   • Dysphonia.[2]
   • Deafness.
   • Dementia.

   1. Aphasia refers to the complete absence of speech.
   2. Due to injury of recurrent laryngeal nerve(s), e.g. following thyroidectomy.

Q6.12 What is the difference between dysphasia and dysarthria?

A: Dysphasia refers to an inability to find words for speech or writing (motor or expressive dysphasia) or to understand them (sensory dysphasia). Dysphasia results from cortical damage. Dysarthria refers to a disturbance of the motor act of speaking, i.e. with the peripheral organs of speech production.

Q6.13 If you suspect that someone has dysphasia or aphasia what other disability will normally be present?

A: A right-sided hemiparesis or hemiplegia.

Q6.14 What are the more common causes of dysarthria?

A:
- Bulbar or pseudobulbar palsy.
- Cerebellar dysarthria.
- Extrapyramidal dysarthria in, for example, parkinsonism.
- Facial nerve palsy.

Q6.15 What should be looked for on examination of the skull?

A:
- Any abnormality in size or shape.
- Local or diffuse swelling(s).
- Nasal or aural discharge.
- Bruits over orbits and carotid arteries (if indicated).

Q6.16 What are the signs of meningeal irritation?

A:
- Neck stiffness.
- Positive Kernig's sign.
- Positive Brudzinski's sign.[1]

1. When the head is flexed, the thighs and knees also flex.

EXAMINATION: CRANIAL NERVES

THE FIRST CRANIAL NERVE (OLFACTORY)

Q6.17 How do you test for evidence of anosmia (Loss of sense or smell)?

A: By testing each nostril separately using well recognized odours.[1]

1. The olfactory nerve is not generally tested during routine neurological examination.

Q6.18 Lesions of the olfactory nerve are uncommon. Name three conditions which may be associated with this problem

A: 1. Tumours, e.g. meningioma or tumour of frontal lobes.

2. Skull fracture.
3. Kallmann's syndrome.*

* Isolated gonadotrophin deficiency associated with anosmia and colour blindness.

THE SECOND CRANIAL NERVE (OPTIC)

Q6.19 What vital functions are served by the optic nerve?

A: • Visual acuity.
   • Fields of vision.
   • Colour vision.[1]

1. Not tested routinely.

Q6.20 Visual acuity is normally tested in each eye separately by the use of Snellen's charts. **How may visual acuity be tested at the bedside?**

A: By using the following clinical standards of vision:[1]

   • Perception of light.
   • Recognition of movement, e.g. movement of fingers.
   • Ability to count fingers.
   • Ability to read large newsprint.
   • Ability to read small newsprint.

   1. If patient is wearing glasses visual acuity should be checked with glasses on.

Q6.21 How do you assess visual fields?

A: • By the confrontation method.
   • By the menace reflex.

Q6.22 What is the menace reflex?

A: In patients who are drowsy or unable to cooperate with the confrontation method, the examiner's hand may be brought rapidly in front of the patient's eye from outside the lateral field of vision. Reflex blinking may be seen as the hand passes in front of the eye.

Q6.23 What is the probable site of the lesion in patients with the following visual field abnormalities?:

1. *Total visual loss in one eye.*
2. *Bitemporal hemianopia.*
3. *Right homonymous hemianopia.*
4. *Homonymous hemianopia with macular sparing.*
5. *Enlarged blind spot.*
6. *Concentric constriction of visual field.*

A: 1. Retina or optic nerve.
    2. Optic chiasma.
    3. Left optic tract.
    4. Optic radiation in posterior part of parietal lobes.
    5. Early papilloedema.
    6. Late papilloedema.

Eyes

General examination

Q6.24 What abnormalities may be seen in the eyes of patients with diffuse toxic goitre (Graves' disease)?

A: • Lid retraction.
    • Lid lag.
    • Exophthalmos.
    • Ophthalmopathy (ophthalmoplegia).

Q6.25 An exophthalmometer should be used to assess accurately the degree of exophthalmos. **How, clinically, are lid retraction and exophthalmos defined?**

A: Lid retraction is present when a rim of sclera can be seen above the iris. Exophthalmos is recognized by the presence of a rim of sclera below the iris.

Q6.26 Does unilateral exophthalmos occur in diffuse toxic goitre?

A: Yes, but in patients with unilateral exophthalmos or proptosis other causes should be considered.

Q6.27 What conditions may cause unilateral proptosis?

A:
- Retro-orbital neoplasms.
- Infections.
- Carotid – cavernous fistulae.[1]

1. If suspected listen over the closed eye for a bruit.

Eyelids
Q6.28 What abnormalities may be seen in the eyelids?

A:
- Ectropion.[1]
- Entropion.[2]
- Hordeolum or stye.[3]
- Chalazion.[4]
- Small follicles on undersurface of upper eyelids in trachoma.
- Periorbital and lid oedema.[5]
- Xanthelasma.[6]
- Lid retraction.
- Ptosis.

1. Common in elderly but may be seen in chronic facial nerve palsy as in Bell's palsy or leprosy.
2. An important sign of trachoma.
3. Infection around eyelash.
4. Swelling caused by obstruction of meibomian glands.
5. May be due to cardiac failure, nephrotic syndrome, drug reaction, hypothyroidism and infection (pyogenic, trichiniasis).
6. Cholesterol deposits which may occur in diabetes mellitus, primary biliary cirrhosis, the nephrotic syndrome and hypercholesterolaemia.

Q6.29 What are the causes of ptosis?

A:
- Palsy of the third cranial nerve.
- Horner's syndrome.
- Muscle disease, e.g. myasthenia gravis.

Conjunctiva

Q6.30 What abnormalities may be seen in the conjunctiva in developed and developing countries?

A: • Conjunctivitis.[1]
   • Chemosis or oedema of the conjunctiva.[2]
   • Bitot's spots with conjunctival pigmentation.[3]
   • Dullness, dryness and wrinkling of the conjunctiva.[3]

1. May be due to a wide variety of causes: viral, bacterial, allergy, foreign body, etc.
2. May be seen in severe exophthalmos, infections, cavernous sinus thrombosis.
3. Important signs of xerophthalmia.

Sclera

Q6.31 What abnormalities may be seen on examination of the sclera?

A: • Jaundice.
   • Blue discoloration.[1]
   • Scleritis.[2]

1. May be seen in iron deficiency anaemia and osteogenesis imperfecta.
2. May rarely be seen in rheumatoid arthritis.

Iris

Q6.32 What will you observe in an acute iritis?

A: Dilatation of ciliary blood vessels, especially around the corneal margin.

Q6.33 What common systemic diseases may be associated with iritis?

A: • Gonorrhoea.
   • Non-specific urethritis.
   • Rheumatoid arthritis.
   • Leprosy.

Cornea

Q6.34 What abnormalities of the cornea should be looked for in developed and developing countries?

A: • Keratitis.[1]
• Corneal ulceration.
• Arcus cornealis (arcus senilis).[2]
• Dullness and dryness (xerosis) of the cornea.[3]
• Corneal softening and bulging of the cornea.[3]
• Greyish film (pannus) over the cornea.[4]

1. Refers to inflammation of the cornea of which there are many different types and causes.
2. A white ring around outer margin of the cornea.
3. Important signs of xerophthalmia and trachoma.
4. An important sign of trachoma, seen at first over the upper part of the cornea.

Pupils

Q6.35 What features should be noted on examination of the pupils?

A: • Size.
• Shape.
• Symmetry.
• Reactivity to light[1] and accommodation.

1. Both direct and consensual reactions should be tested.

Q6.36 Which nerve fibres cause constriction of the pupil?

A: Parasympathetic nerve fibres which enter the orbit in association with the third cranial nerve (oculomotor).

Q6.37 Which fibres cause dilatation of the pupil?

A: Sympathetic nerve fibres from the superior cervical ganglion.

Q6.38 Why is the pupil dilated in a palsy of the third cranial nerve?

A: Because parasympathetic pupillary constricting fibres run in association with the third cranial nerve.

Q6.39 Why is the pupil constricted in Horner's syndrome?

A: Because Horner's syndrome results, usually, from a lesion of the cervical sympathetic chain.

Q6.40 When you test the light reflex what are the afferent and efferent parts of the reflex?

A: The afferent impulses are carried by the optic nerve and the efferent impulses by the parasympathetic fibres, which enter the orbit in association with the third cranial nerve.

Q6.41 If you test the light reflex in an eye with a third nerve palsy, what will you observe?

A: Loss of direct light reaction but preservation of consensual light reaction.

Q6.42 Do you understand why?

A: Yes, the efferent part of the light reflex is lost in the affected eye but present in the normal eye.

Q6.43 If you have a patient with an optic nerve lesion in one eye, and the other eye is normal, what will you observe if you test the light reflex in the normal eye?

A: Direct light reaction will be observed in the normal eye and consensual light reaction in the affected eye.

Q6.44 If you test the light reflex in the eye with the optic nerve lesion, what will you observe?

A: Loss of direct and consensual light reactions.

Q6.45 How do you test the convergence (accommodation) reflex?

A: Ask the patient to relax accommodation by looking at the ceiling or a distant object. Ask him or her then to look at a pen held close to the nose. As he or she looks at the pen the eyes converge and the pupils constrict.

Q6.46 What are Argyll Robertson pupils?

A: Small and irregular pupils which react to accommodation but not to light.

Q6.47 What are Holmes–Adie pupils?

A: Large dilated pupils[1] which react sluggishly to both light and accommodation. They may be associated with absent reflexes.

1. May be unilateral.

Q6.48 In what conditions can you see bilateral constricted pupils (miosis)?

A: • Opiate use.
   • Pilocarpine and other parasympathetic stimulatory drugs.
   • Iritis.
   • Corneal and conjunctival irritation.
   • Lesions in the pons.

Q6.49 In what conditions can you see dilated pupils?

A: • Anxiety.
   • Use of mydriatic drops, e.g. atropine.
   • Holmes–Adie pupils.[1]
   • A third cranial nerve lesion.[1]
   • Acute glaucoma.[1]
   • Damage to the optic nerve.[1]

1. May be or usually unilateral.

Q6.50 Describe the features of a third cranial nerve palsy

A: • Ptosis.
   • Dilatation of pupil.
   • The affected eye will be deviated outwards and downwards.
   • Absent pupillary reflexes.

Q6.51 Describe the features of Horner's syndrome.[1]

A: • Constriction of the pupil.
• Ptosis.
• Ipsilateral anhidrosis.
• Enophthalmos.

1. All features may not be present.

Eye Movements
Q6.52 What is meant by conjugate gaze?

A: • Conjugate gaze refers to the normal linked parallel movements of the eyes that are controlled by complex upper motor neurone mechanisms. Brain lesions may lead to failure of conjugate lateral and vertical gaze. The latter is associated with upper brainstem lesions.

THE OCULOMOTOR (THIRD), TROCHLEAR (FOURTH) AND ABDUCENS (SIXTH) CRANIAL NERVES

Q6.53 What must you ask patients whom you suspect may have a palsy of cranial nerves III, IV and VI?

A: If they have diplopia, and if the answer is 'yes', in what direction diplopia is maximal.

Q6.54 What procedures must you adopt when testing eye movements?

A: • Hold the patient's head steady with one hand using the other to test eye movements with a moving target such as a pen.
• The pen should be held approximately 50 cm (18 inches) from the patient's eyes.
• Movement should be tested in vertical and horizontal planes.

Q6.55 Which external ocular muscles are supplied by the oculomotor (third) nerve?

A: Levator palpebrae superioris, the superior, medial and inferior recti, and the inferior oblique muscles.

Q6.56 Which muscle is supplied by the trochlear (fourth) nerve?

A: The superior oblique muscle.

Q6.57 Which muscle is supplied by the abducens (sixth) nerve?

A: The lateral rectus muscle.

Q6.58 Which other nerve fibres accompany the third cranial nerve?

A: Preganglionic parasympathetic nerve fibres which run to the ciliary ganglion, from where postganglionic fibres supply the sphincter of the pupil.

Q6.59 Which nerve fibres cause dilatation of the pupil?

A: Postganglionic sympathetic nerve fibres from the superior cervical ganglion.

Q6.60 Which muscle(s) is responsible for turning the eye outwards (abduction)?

A: The lateral rectus.

Q6.61 Which muscle(s) is responsible for turning the eye inwards (adduction)?

A: The medial rectus.

Q6.62 Which muscle(s) is responsible for turning the eye upwards with the eye in the mid-position?

A: The inferior oblique and superior rectus.

Q6.63 Which muscle(s) is responsible for turning the eye downwards with the eye in the mid-position?

A: The superior oblique and inferior rectus.

Q6.64 While testing eye movements what else should be looked for?

A: Nystagmus.

Q6.65 How is nystagmus classified according to its appearance?

A: • Phasic or jerky nystagmus where oscillations have a quick and slow component in a linear plane.
   • Rotary or pendular nystagmus, where oscillations occur in a two-dimensional plane along the arc of a circle.

Q6.66 What does phasic nystagmus usually indicate?

A: A lesion of the eighth cranial nerve, the vestibular pathways or cerebellum. It may also be seen in heavy drinkers.

Q6.67 With what is rotary nystagmus associated?

A: Defective vision, for example, in albinism.

Ophthalmoscopy

Q6.68 Ophthalmoscopy is a technique with which every medical student should be familiar. Your patient's life may depend upon your ability to use an ophthalmoscope. **What does the number of each lens indicate?**

A: Its focal length expressed in dioptres.

Q6.69 What is the shape of ' + ' lenses?

A: Convex.

Q6.70 What is the shape of ' − ' lenses?

A: Concave.

Q6.71 Ophthalmoscopy is best conducted in a darkened room. **If a thorough examination of the fundus is required, what must you do?**

A: Dilate the pupils with a mydriatic solution, e.g. tropicamide or cyclopentolate hydrochloride.

Q6.72 After examination is completed what should be done?[1]

A: Pupils should be constricted with 1% pilocarpine or 2% eserine sulphate drops.

1. Probably not always necessary.

Q6.73 If a ' + ' lens is required to see the fundus clearly, what does this indicate?

A: Hypermetropia.

Q6.74 If a ' − ' lens is required what does this indicate?

A: Myopia.[1]

1. In a very myopic eye a − 20 lens may be required.

Q6.75 What are the main causes or absence of the red reflex?

A: • Cataract.
    • Vitreous haemorrhage.
    • Retinal detachment.

Q6.76 In examination of the fundi what should be checked systematically?

A: • The optic discs, their size, shape, colour, margins and physiological cup.
    • Blood vessels, especially their calibre and tortuosity, and arteriovenous crossings.[1]
    • Retina for exudates, haemorrhages, new vessels and pigmentary abnormalities.
    • Macula and fovea.[2]

1. The artery lies on top of the vein and the column of blood should not be altered at the point of crossing.
2. The macula is best viewed by asking patient to look at the light of the ophthalmoscope. The normal macula is darker in colour and free of blood vessels. It is situated about 2 disc diameters to the temporal side of the optic disc.

Q6.77 What fundal changes are seen in papilloedema and papillitis?[1]

A: • Hyperaemia of the disc.
   • Loss of the disc margins.
   • Obliteration of the physiological cup.
   • Congestion and dilatation of veins and loss of pulsation.
   • Haemorrhages radiating from the disc.

   1. Papillitis is secondary to an intrinsic lesion of the optic nerve.

Q6.78 What fundal changes may be seen in hypertension?

A: • Tortuous arteries ⎫
   • Arteriovenous nipping ⎬ grades I and II
   • Varying calibre of the vessels ⎭
   • Flame-shaped haemorrhages ⎫ grade III
   • Hard exudates ⎭
   • Papilloedema – grade IV

Q6.79 How is diabetic retinopathy classified?

A: • Background retinopathy[1] marked by venous dilatation and tortuosity, microaneurysms, blot haemorrhages and soft (cotton-wool) exudates.
   • Maculopathy characterized by macular oedema,[2] exudates and haemorrhages around the macula.
   • Proliferative retinopathy characterized by new vessel formation, vitreous haemorrhage, retinal detachment and retinitis proliferans.

   1. Background retinopathy can progress to either maculopathy or proliferative retinopathy.
   2. May be very difficult to detect by the non-expert.

THE FIFTH CRANIAL NERVE (TRIGEMINAL)

Q6.80 The fifth cranial nerve has both motor and sensory divisions. **What are the three branches of the sensory division?**

A: The ophthalmic, maxillary and mandibular branches.

Q6.81 What are the main muscles supplied by the motor division of the trigeminal nerve?

A: The pterygoid, temporalis and masseter muscles.

Q6.82 How do you test the fifth cranial nerve?

A: 1. Sensation: Light touch and pain (pinprick) sensation is tested on each side of the forehead, cheeks and jaws.
   2. The corneal reflex in which the cornea is touched carefully with a wisp of cotton wool. The efferent impulses of the reflex are carried in the seventh cranial nerve.
   3. Motor function:
      (i) masseters: palpate the masseters as the patient clenches his teeth.
      (ii) pterygoids: ask the patient to open and close the jaw against resistance. In a fifth nerve lesion the jaw will move towards the side of the lesion.
   4. Jaw jerk: In a bilateral upper motor neurone lesion the jaw jerk is brisk.

THE SEVENTH CRANIAL NERVE (FACIAL)

Q6.83 The seventh cranial nerve supplies all the facial muscles except the levator palpebrae superioris. **During its course in the facial canal describe its major anatomical features**

A: • It 'develops' a swelling known as the geniculate ganglion which is joined by the pars intermedia, and the greater superficial and lesser superficial petrosal nerves.
    • Below the geniculate ganglion it gives off the nerve to the stapedius and is joined by the chorda tympani.

Q6.84 What is the function of the chorda tympani?

A: It transmits taste sensation from the anterior two-thirds of the tongue.

Q6.85 Taste sensation from the posterior one-third of the tongue is transmitted via which cranial nerve?

A: The glossopharyngeal nerve.

Q6.86 What are the four fundamental tastes?

A: Sweet, sour, bitter and salt.

Q6.87 Taste is not tested routinely, but if loss of sensation is found over the anterior two-thirds of the tongue in association with a lower motor neurone lesion of the seventh cranial nerve, where is the lesion likely to be?

A: In the facial canal.

Q6.88 What does a lesion involving the nerve to stapedius cause?

A: Hyperacusis.

Q6.89 How should you test the facial muscles?

A: Ask the patient to:
- wrinkle the forehead;
- close the eyes;[1]
- puff out the cheeks;
- show the teeth (not smile);
- whistle.

1. As well as asking the patient to voluntarily close the eyes, lesser degrees of weakness can be detected by trying to open the eyes against resistance with the thumbs of both hands.

Q6.90 With what is an upper motor neurone lesion of the seventh cranial nerve almost always associated?

A: A hemiplegia.

Q6.91 How do you distinguish between a unilateral upper and lower motor neurone lesion of the seventh cranial nerve?

A: In a lower motor neurone lesion all the facial muscles are weak or paralysed on the affected side, whilst in an upper motor neurone lesion the frontalis and orbicularis oculi muscles are spared, i.e. the paralysis affects only the muscles of the lower half of the face.

Q6.92 What are the main causes of a lower motor neurone lesion of the seventh cranial nerve?

A:
- Bell's palsy.
- Leprosy.

Q6.93 What is the Ramsay-Hunt syndrome?

A: Involvement of the geniculate ganglion, usually by the herpes zoster virus. The features of the syndrome are:
- A lower motor neurone facial palsy.
- Loss of taste over the anterior two-thirds of the tongue (same side as the lesion).
- Herpes vesicles around the external auditory meatus, and sometimes over the ipsilateral fauces.
- Pain around the ear which may precede the appearance of vesicles.

THE EIGHTH CRANIAL NERVE (VESTIBULOCOCHLEAR)

Q6.94 The eighth cranial nerve has two components: the cochlear and vestibular division. **How do you test the cochlear (auditory) division at the bedside?**

A:
- Test each ear separately by whispering numbers, or by holding a ticking watch close to each ear. The ear not being tested should be occluded by a finger.
- By performing Rinne's test and Weber's test to help determine if deafness is due to a lesion within the external auditory meatus or middle ear (conduction deafness), or to a lesion affecting the cochlea or its nerve (perception or nerve deafness).

Q6.95 What is Rinne's test?

A: In Rinne's test a vibrating tuning fork is held initially near the ear and then over the mastoid process until the sound disappears. It is then held close to the external auditory meatus. If the sound is heard again, as it is normally, nerve deafness is likely. Air conduction is louder than bone conduction in normal subjects and in patients with nerve deafness, whilst bone conduction is louder in conduction deafness.

Q6.96 What is Weber's test?

A: In Weber's test the vibrating tuning fork is held in the middle of the patient's forehead. If the sound is referred to the good ear it indicates nerve deafness in the opposite ear whilst if referred to the deaf ear it indicates middle ear deafness. In normal hearing the sound is heard in the mid-line.

Q6.97 Are Rinne's and Weber's tests always reliable?

A: No, patients with deafness should have audiometry.

Q6.98 What symptoms result from damage to the cochlear division of the eighth cranial nerve?

A: • Diminished hearing.
   • Tinnitus.

Q6.99 Can vestibular function be tested easily at the bedside?

A: No, but the presence or absence of nystagmus will have been noted on examination of eye movements.

Q6.100 What symptom results from damage to the vestibular division of the eighth cranial nerve?

A: Vertigo.

THE NINTH CRANIAL NERVE (GLOSSOPHARYNGEAL) AND
TENTH CRANIAL NERVE (VAGUS)

Q6.101 The glossopharyngeal nerve is a mixed motor and
sensory nerve. Many of its functions are associated with those
of the tenth cranial nerve (the vagus) which is also a mixed
nerve. **How is the combined motor function of these two
nerves normally tested?**

A: By asking the patient to say 'Ah' and watching palatal
movement. In a normal person the palate should rise in
the mid-line. In a bilateral palsy therefore the palate will
not move, or only partially move, and in a unilateral palsy
the palate and uvula will be pulled away from the weak
side.

**Q6.102 Which reflexes are sometimes elicited in testing
the sensory function of the glossopharyngeal nerve, and
motor function of the vagus?**

A: The gag reflex[1] in which the posterior wall of the
pharynx is touched by a tongue depressor, and the palatal
reflex in which each side of the palate is touched by a little
stick or similar instrument.

1. This is unpleasant for the patient and should not be
carried out routinely.

Q6.103 How can a lesion of the vagus affect speech?

A: • By involvement of its recurrent laryngeal branch which
will cause dysphonia.
• By paralysis of the palate which will give a nasal quality
to speech.

THE ELEVENTH CRANIAL NERVE (THE SPINAL
ACCESSORY NERVE)

Q6.104 How is the accessory nerve tested?

A: By assessing the power of the sternomastoid[1] and tra-
pezius muscles against resistance.[2]

1. The patient is first asked to press the chin down against resistance, and then to turn the head against resistance to each side in turn.
2. The patient is asked to shrug the shoulders. Evidence of wasting should also be looked for.

Q6.105 Are you ever likely to see a unilateral upper motor neurone lesion of cranial nerves IX, X and XI?

A: No, since all have bilateral cerebral representation.

THE TWELFTH CRANIAL NERVE (THE HYPOGLOSSAL)

Q6.106 What are the signs of a lower motor lesion of the tongue?

A: • Fasciculation.
    • Wasting.
    • Deviation of the tongue on protrusion towards the affected side in a unilateral lesion of the hypoglossal nerve.

Q6.107 What are the signs of a bilateral upper motor neurone lesion of the tongue?

A: A relatively immobile, spastic tongue.[1]

1. This usually occurs as part of a pseudobulbar palsy.

Q6.108 Are you ever likely to see a unilateral upper motor neurone lesion of the hypoglossal nerve?

A: Very rarely, and only in association with an upper motor neurone lesion of the arm and leg (hemiplegia).

Q6.109 In what condition may rapid protrusion and retraction of the tongue be seen?

A: Parkinsonism.

Q6.110 What are 'bulbar' palsies?

A: Bulbar palsies are labioglossopalatopharyngeal palsies.

Q6.111 What is the difference between a pseudobulbar palsy and a bulbar palsy?

A: A pseudobulbar palsy is a supranuclear or upper motor neurone lesion of muscles supplied by cranial nerves IX, X, XI and XII and sometimes by cranial nerves V and VII whilst a bulbar palsy is a bilateral lower motor neurone lesion of muscles supplied by the same cranial nerves.

Q6.112 What is the main cause of a pseudobulbar palsy?

A: Vascular lesions in both internal capsules.

Q6.113 What are the signs of a pseudobulbar palsy?

A: • Dysarthria.
   • Dysphonia.
   • Dysphagia.[1]
   • Spastic immobile tongue.
   • Brisk jaw jerk.

   1. Worse with fluids.

Q6.114 What are the signs of a bulbar palsy?

A: • Dysarthria.
   • Dysphonia.
   • Dysphagia.
   • Bilateral wasting and fasciculation of the tongue.
   • Paralysis of the palate.

Q6.115 What are the main causes of a bulbar palsy?

A: • Motor neurone disease.
   • Poliomyelitis.
   • Acute ascending polyneuritis.
   • Lead poisoning.
   • Botulism.

Q6.116 How do you test for evidence of nerve root irritation when lumbar or sacral nerve roots are involved?

A: By straight leg raising, i.e. by flexing the hip with the knee straight.

INVOLUNTARY MOVEMENTS

Q6.117 What kinds of involuntary movements may be seen in clinical practice?

A:
- Tremors.
- Choreiform movements.[1]
- Athetoid movements.[2]
- Tics.[3]

1. Choreiform movements are 'involuntary, abrupt, jerky and of short duration'.
2. Athetoid movements are involuntary, slow, sinuous, writhing, twisting movements.
3. Repetitive involuntary movements usually involving one group of muscles, e.g. facial grimacing.

TREMOR

Q6.118 What are some of the different types of tremor that may be seen on clinical examination?

A:
- The fine or physiological tremor which is seen in anxiety, thyrotoxicosis, alcoholism, and with certain drugs.[1]
- The coarse tremor at rest of Parkinson's disease, the 'pill-rolling' tremor.[2]
- Asterixis or flapping tremor seen in hepatic failure.
- Benign essential tremor seen most commonly in the elderly.
- Intention tremor of cerebellar disease not present at rest, but which appears on movement and is most noticeable towards the end of a voluntary movement.

1. Tricyclic antidepressants, phenothiazines, reserpine, anticonvulsants.
2. The tremor of Parkinson's disease disappears during sleep and is aggravated by emotion and fine movements.

MUSCLE WEAKNESS

Q6.119 When confronted by weakness or paralysis of one or more limbs what question must you ask yourself?

A: Is the paralysis due to an upper or a lower motor neurone lesion?

Q6.120 What is meant by an upper motor neurone (UMN) lesion?

A: A lesion involving the pyramidal tracts (corticospinal tracts).

Q6.121 What are the features of an upper motor neurone lesion?

A: • Muscle weakness.
- Extensor plantar response.
- Hyperreflexia of tendon reflexes.
- Sustained clonus.
- Diminution or absence of abdominal reflexes.
- Increased tone (spasticity) of 'clasp-knife' type.
- No muscle wasting.

Q6.122 What is meant by a lower motor neurone (LMN) lesion?

A: A lesion caused by involvement of the motor pathway from the anterior horn cells or equivalent cells in the brainstem to the neuromuscular junction. (Some would also include muscle disease as part of lower motor neurone lesions, but in muscle disease the reflexes are usually present until the disease is far advanced.)

Q6.123 What are the features of a lower motor neurone lesion?

A: • Muscle weakness.
- Wasting.
- Reduced tone (hypotonicity, flaccidity).
- Diminished or absent reflexes.
- Involuntary movements (fasciculation).

Q6.124 Is it usually easy to distinguish between an upper and a lower motor neurone lesion?

A: Yes, but sometimes a mixed picture may be seen, for example, in motor neurone disease. Sometimes also all the classic features may not be present, e.g. tone may sometimes be decreased following a stroke.

TESTING MUSCLE POWER

Q6.125 Power in the upper limbs should be examined systematically. **How would you test muscle power in an orderly way in the hands and arms?** As you test think 'Which movement am I testing?', 'Which muscle(s) am I testing?', 'Which nerve am I testing?' and 'Which spinal segments am I testing?' (Often during examination students ask the patient to grip fingers, or raise the leg without a clear understanding of what they are testing. During routine examination it is quite impracticable to test every muscle and nerve. The following scheme for examination of power in the upper and lower limbs will ensure that little of importance is missed.)

A:

	Movement	Muscle[1]	Nerve	Spinal segment[2]
In the hand				
Little finger	Abduction	Abductor digiti minimi	Ulnar	C8 T1
Thumb	Abduction	Abductor pollicis brevis	Median	C8 T1
Four fingers	Extension of MP joints	Extensor digitorum	Radial	C7 C8
In the arm				
Wrist	Extension	Extensor carpi radialis longus	Radial	C5 C6
		Extensor carpi ulnaris	Radial	C7 C8
	Flexion	Flexor carpi radialis	Median	C6 C7
		Flexor carpi ulnaris	Ulnar	C7 C8 T1
Elbow	Extension	Triceps	Radial	C6 C7 C8
	Flexion	Biceps	Musculo-cutaneous	C5 C6
Shoulder	Abduction	Supraspinatus	Supra-scapular	C5 C6
		Deltoid	Circumflex	C5 C6

[1] It is probably not necessary to remember names of all the muscles.
[2] Underlining indicates most important spinal segments from which nerve is derived.

Q6.126 Power in the lower limbs should be examined systematically. How would you test muscle power in the legs?

A:

	Movement	Muscle[1]	Nerve	Spinal segment[2]
Hip	Extension	Gluteus maximus	Sciatic	L5 S1 S2
	Flexion	Iliopsoas	Femoral	L1 L2 L3
Knee	Extension	Quadriceps femoris	Femoral	L2 L3 L4
	Flexion	Hamstrings	Sciatic	L5 S1 S2
Ankle	Dorsiflexion	Tibialis anterior	Sciatic (deep peroneal)	L4 L5
	Plantar flexion	Gastrocnemius	Sciatic (tibial)	S1 S2
Foot	Inversion	Tibialis posterior	Sciatic (tibial)	L4 L5
	Eversion	Peroneus longus and brevis	Sciatic (superior peroneal)	L5 S1

[1] It is probably not necessary to remember names of all the muscles.

[2] Underlining indicates most important spinal segments from which nerve is derived.

RECORDING OF MUSCLE POWER

Q6.127 Describe the scale used for recording muscle power

A: 0. No contraction.
1. Flicker or trace of contraction.
2. Active movement, with gravity eliminated.
3. Active movement against gravity.
4. Active movement against gravity and resistance.*
5. Normal power.

   * Grade 4 is sometimes subdivided into grades 4 −, 4 and 4 + to indicate movement against slight, moderate and strong resistance respectively.

MUSCLE TONE

Q6.128 Describe the variations in muscle tone that you could encounter?

A: • Increased tone or spasticity ('clasp-knife') in an upper motor neurone lesion.

- Increased tone or rigidity in parkinsonism ('lead pipe' or 'cog-wheel').
- Decreased tone (hypotonia) in lower motor neurone lesions and following an acute upper motor neurone lesion.

REFLEXES

Q6.129 How are reflexes classified?

A: Into tendon and superficial (cutaneous) reflexes.

TENDON REFLEXES

Q6.130 Name the common tendon reflexes and their corresponding spinal segments

A: 1. Supinator   C6
   2. Biceps   C5
   3. Triceps   C6 C7
   4. Knee   L3 L4
   5. Ankle   L5 S1

Q6.131 What is the main cause of increased tendon reflexes?

A: An upper motor neurone lesion, but brisk reflexes can also be observed in anxious patients, and in hepatic coma and uraemia.

Q6.132 What causes diminished or absent reflexes?

A: A lower motor neurone lesion, although in some normal people reflexes may be difficult to elicit. Diminished reflexes may also be found after severe upper motor neurone damage.

Q6.133 In a patient in whom you find absent knee or ankle reflexes, what should be done to confirm your findings?

A: Reinforcement, in which the patient is asked to hook both hands together then to pull forcibly without letting the fingers go.

Q6.134 If you find absent reflexes in the upper limbs how could you carry out reinforcement?

A: By asking the patient to clench the jaws or push both knees together.

SUPERFICIAL REFLEXES

Q6.135 What are the main superficial reflexes?

A: 1. The plantar reflex   L5, S1
   2. Abdominal reflexes

THE PLANTAR REFLEX

Q6.136 What is the special value of the plantar reflex?

A: It is of great value in the identification of an upper motor neurone lesion. (In tropical neurology the plantar reflexes may be difficult to elicit in patients either with or without an upper motor neurone lesion.)

Q6.137 What happens in a upper motor neurone lesion when you elicit the plantar reflex?

A: There is dorsiflexion of the great toe accompanied usually by a spreading of the other four toes (Babinski's sign).

ABDOMINAL REFLEXES

Q6.138 Do absent abdominal reflexes usually indicate an upper or a lower motor neurone lesion?

A: An upper motor neurone lesion.

Q6.139 What else may be associated with absent abdominal reflexes?

A: Obesity or a lax abdominal wall in multiparous women.

Q6.140 Is an extensor plantar response always associated with brisk reflexes?

A: Yes, usually, but in subacute combined degeneration of the cord, and motor neurone disease, you may find an extensor plantar response in association with absent knee and ankle jerks.

COORDINATION

Q6.141 In which two conditions is incoordination an important feature?[1]

A: • Sensory ataxia that results from defective proprioception.
   • Cerebellar ataxia.

   1. Weakness of muscles may also be associated with clumsy or awkward movement.

Q6.142 Which tests are used in the detection of incoordination?

A: The finger–nose test and the heel–knee test.

Q6.143 How can you distinguish between incoordination due to sensory ataxia and cerebellar ataxia using these two tests?

A: The patient with sensory ataxia will perform the tests better with the eyes open, whilst the patient with cerebellar ataxia will perform equally badly with the eyes open or closed.

Q6.144 In cerebellar ataxia, what will also be observed during the finger–nose test as part of the general picture of incoordination?

A: Intention tremor – as the patient's finger approaches the nose movements become more clumsy, and he may overshoot the nose.

Q6.145 What is dysdiadochokinesia?

A: One manifestation of ataxia in cerebellar disease. It is seen when the patient is asked to perform rapid alternating movements such as pronating and supinating the forearm as quickly as possible.

SENSATION

Q6.146 What different sensations are tested when testing the sensory system?

A: • Light touch with a piece of cotton wool.
   • Pain.
   • Joint position sense.
   • Deep pain (muscle and tendon sense).
   • Vibration.
   • Temperature.[1]

   1. Temperature is usually not tested routinely but temperature testing may be very valuable in leprosy where temperature sense is lost early.

Q6.147 Name the different kinds of sensory loss that may be encountered in patients with neurological disease

A: • 'Glove and stocking' or symmetrical and distal sensory loss in peripheral neuropathy, e.g. diabetes mellitus or thiamine deficiency.
   • Sensory loss in specific areas supplied by one or more peripheral nerve(s), e.g. in leprosy you often find sensory loss in the area of the hand supplied by the ulnar nerve.
   • Sensory loss over specific dermatomes associated with nerve root lesions.
   • Sensory loss associated with brain and spinal cord lesions.

Q6.148 Over which part of the hand is the ulnar nerve responsible for sensation?

A: Over the little finger and one half of the ring finger.

Q6.149 Describe the dermatomes of the lower limbs

A:
- Inguinal   L1
- Anterior thigh   L2, L3
- Shin   L4, L5
- Lateral border of foot, sole and back of calf   S1

Q6.150 What sensory modalities will be lost in a lesion of the posterior or dorsal columns?

A: Loss of joint, vibration and deep pain (muscle and tendon sense).

Q6.151 List all the signs that may be found in a posterior column lesion

A:
- Loss of joint position sense, vibration and deep pain.
- Ataxia with eyes closed (positive Romberg's sign) and disturbance of gait.
- Diminution of deep reflexes.
- Hypotonicity.

Q6.152 In a patient with selective loss of pain and temperature in both legs, where is the lesion causing this problem located?

A: In the central part of the spinal cord.

Q6.153 If there is unilateral selective loss of pain and temperature where is the lesion almost certainly located?

A: In one of the spinothalamic tracts, in the tract on the opposite side to that of the affected leg.

Q6.154 Describe the neurological findings in a patient with the Brown–Séquard syndrome, i.e. a lesion involving one half of the spinal cord

A:
- Ipsilateral paralysis below the lesion.
- Ipsilateral brisk reflexes.
- Ipsilateral increased tone.

- Ipsilateral sensory loss at the level of the lesion.
- Ipsilateral loss of joint, vibration and deep pain (muscle and tendon sense).
- Contralateral loss of pain and temperature sensation.
- Sphincter disturbances.

Q6.155 How would you test a patient with suspected damage to the sensory cortex?

A:
- Two-point discrimination.
- Stereognosis in which patient is asked to identify objects by palpation.
- Sensory inattention or extinction.[1]

1. Refers to an inability to recognize that both legs are being touched at once, whilst the patient can identify each leg correctly when touched in succession.

CEREBELLAR DISEASE

Q6.156 What are the main features of cerebellar disease?

A:
- Nystagmus.[1]
- Dysarthria.
- Intention tremor.
- Ataxia.
- Hypotonicity of limbs.[2]
- Pendular reflexes.[2]

1. Coarse and jerking.
2. Often difficult to demonstrate.

Q6.157 What are some of the more common causes of cerebellar disease?

A:
- Drugs – alcohol, phenytoin.
- Neoplasm.
- Hypothyroidism.
- Friedreich's ataxia.
- Degenerative disease.

Q6.158 How may ataxia be looked for?

A: • By inspection of gait.
   • By testing coordination in upper limbs.
   • By testing coordination in lower limbs.

Q6.159 What is an intention tremor?

A: A tremor that increases in amplitude as the hand reaches the target.

Q6.160 In a patient with an ataxic gait, what two main causes of the ataxia should be considered?

A: 1. Cerebellar disease.
   2. Sensory ataxia due to a posterior column lesion or severe peripheral neuropathy, e.g. in diabetes mellitus.

Q6.161 How may you distinguish between these two causes by observation of the patient's gait?

A: • The patient with cerebellar ataxia may look ahead whilst the patient with sensory ataxia often looks to the floor, since sensory ataxia can be reduced by visual information. In cerebellar ataxia visual information makes no difference.
   • Romberg's test – in sensory ataxia Romberg's test is positive. If the patient stands with his feet together and closes his eyes he will sway and tend to fall. In cerebellar disease the patient tends to sway or fall towards the side of the lesion.

Q6.162 Apart from patients with an ataxic gait due to cerebellar disease or sensory ataxia, what other abnormal gaits are commonly seen in clinical practice?

A: • A hemiplegic gait – the patient walks with an extended leg and flexed arm.

- A paraplegic (scissor) gait – the patient displays marked stiffness of both legs with the feet remaining on the ground.
- The shuffling, festinating gait of Parkinson's disease. The patient also walks with a stooped posture.
- The high-stepping gait associated with a lateral popliteal nerve palsy. The patient displays foot drop, a high lift and tendency for the affected foot to slap down on the floor.
- A waddling gait in which the hips are alternately tilted. Seen in patients with proximal myopathies and limb–girdle muscular dystrophy.

Q6.163 What are the main features of extrapyramidal lesions?

A:
- Involuntary movements.[1]
- Increase in muscle tone.[2]
- Bradykinesia, akinesia.[3]

1. Usually coarse 'pill-rolling' tremor but may be choreiform or athetoid.
2. Jerky (cog-wheel) or uniform (lead-pipe) rigidity.
3. Slowness in starting and performing emotional and voluntary movements.

Q6.164 What are the main clinical features of Parkinson's disease?

A:
- Arhythmic resting tremor.
- Rigidity.
- Bradykinesia.[1]
- Postural defect.[2]

1. Bradykinesia refers to slowness in movement, poverty of movement and loss of normal associated movements such as reduced arm-swing when walking.
2. Patient becomes progressively more stooped.

Q6.165 Now that you have covered the essentials in the examination of the nervous system write down your plan for examination of a patient with neurological disease.

A: Summary plan for examination of a patient with neurological disease

General	Higher cerebral function
	• Level of consciousness
	• Appearance and behaviour
	• Memory and intelligence
	• Mood
	• Presence of hallucinations and delusions
	• Speech
	Examination of skull
	Examination for signs of meningeal irritation
	Examination for signs of nerve root irritation
	Presence of involuntary movements
The cranial nerves	Include examination of pupils and testing for nystagmus
Limbs and trunk	
The motor system	• Weakness of any muscle or muscle group
	• Muscle wasting and fasciculation
	• Muscle tone
Reflexes	• Tendon
	• Superficial including plantar reflex
Coordination	Test with eyes open and closed
Sensory	• Touch
	• Pain
	• Joint position sense
	• Deep pain (muscle and tendon sense)
	• Vibration
	• Temperature
Gait	When the patient is standing test for rombergism
Spine	Examine carefully if evidence of a root or cord lesion

Q6.166 During the routine examination of patients without obvious neurological symptoms is it necessary to follow the scheme for testing the central nervous system described in Q6.165?

A: No, but it is wise during routine examination to ensure that your patient has no evidence of significant neurological disease by making the following observations:

General	Speech and involuntary movements	These will be observed during history taking and examination
	Neck stiffness	Important to check if the patient is febrile or complains of headache
Cranial nerves	Eyes	Ensure that the patient can see with both eyes. Examine the pupils and fundi
	Facial movements	Ask the patient to close his eyes tightly and show his teeth
	Hearing	Ensure that the patient can hear properly
	Tongue	Examine the tongue
Limbs and trunk Motor	Muscle wasting	Inspect the limbs carefully
	Muscle weakness	Ask the patient to stretch out the arms. In the legs check flexion and extension of the knee and dorsiflexion of the ankle
Reflexes	Tendon and superficial	Check the tendon reflexes in the upper and lower limbs, and the plantar reflex
Gait		Observe the patient standing and walking, if possible

7
THE BLOOD

THE HAEMOPOIETIC SYSTEM

HISTORY

Q7.1 Name the non-specific symptoms of anaemia

A: • Tiredness.
   • Breathlessness.
   • Palpitations.
   • Headache.
   • Ankle swelling.
   • Angina and intermittent claudication.[1]

   1. In older patients.

Q7.2 What symptoms can be found in a patient with leukopenia (neutropenia)?

A: • History of recurrent infections.
   • Mouth, throat, anal and skin ulceration.

   1. Infections are predominantly bacterial, but viral, fungal and protozoal infections also occur with increased frequency.

Q7.3 Describe the symptoms which may be associated with a bleeding disorder[1]

A: • Spontaneous bleeding into the skin (purpura).[2,3]
   • Bleeding from the gums or epistaxis.[3]
   • Menorrhagia in women.[3]
   • Excessive bleeding after minor trauma or surgery.[4]

- Pains in joints and muscles.[4]
- Haematuria, gastrointestinal bleeding and intracranial bleeding.[4]

1. Abnormal bleeding may result from vascular disorders, thrombocytopenia, defects in platelet function or disorders of blood coagulation.
2. This may result from acquired vascular defects (senile purpura, purpura associated with infections, steroid therapy, scurvy and the Henoch–Schönlein syndrome) or from platelet disorders. Easy bruising may also be seen in apparently healthy women.
3. Symptoms that are more commonly associated with platelet disorders.
4. Symptoms that are more commonly associated with disorders of coagulation. Bleeding into joints is the most disabling complication of haemophilia.

Q7.4 What other symptoms should be looked for in patients with diseases of the blood?

A:
- Blood in urine, stool and vomitus.
- Menstrual history in females.
- Diarrhoea.[1]
- Abdominal pain.[2]
- Weight loss.[3]
- Fever and sweating.[3]
- Backache.[4]
- Pruritus.[5]

1. Diarrhoea may indicate steatorrhoea and malabsorption. It may also occasionally be associated with pernicious anaemia. In patients with neutropenia diarrhoea may point to intestinal infection.
2. If the spleen is large the patient may complain of a dragging pain in the abdomen.
3. Symptoms associated with leukaemias and lymphomas.
4. Backache is common in patients with multiple myeloma.
5. Pruritus occurs in Hodgkin's disease, chronic lymphatic leukaemia and polycythaemia vera.

SOCIAL/FAMILY/DRUG HISTORY

Q7.5 What points should be noted in the social and family history?

A: • Dietary history.[1]
   • Alcohol intake.[2]
   • Drug intake.[3]
   • Occupation.[4]
   • Family history of bleeding disorders.
   • Travel abroad.[5]
   • Country of origin.[6]
   • Whether pregnant.

1. In developing countries the very young and elderly are at special risk of inadequate dietary intake whilst in developed countries special attention should be paid to the elderly, especially if living alone or disabled.
2. Dietary intake may be inadequate in heavy drinkers, and excess alcohol intake may also be associated with hepatic cirrhosis, portal hypertension and bleeding from the gastrointestinal tract.
3. A wide variety of drugs may cause a wide variety of blood disorders.
4. There may be a history of for example, exposure to chemicals.
5. Patient may have acquired a parasitic infection, e.g. malaria or hookworm.
6. Important when considering disorders such as sickle-cell disease and thalassaemia.

PAST MEDICAL HISTORY

Q7.6 What conditions should be looked for in the past medical history? (Questions asked should relate to the particular problem with which you are faced)

A: • History of blood disease.
   • History of blood transfusions.
   • Excess bleeding after dental extractions.
   • History of fever and recurrent infections.[1]
   • Past history of surgery.[2]

- Jaundice.[3]
- Peptic ulceration.
- Diabetes.[4]
- Chronic respiratory disease.[5]
- Other chronic diseases that may be associated with anaemia, e.g. malignant disease, rheumatoid arthritis, renal failure.

1. Commonly found in B-thalassaemia major, sickle-cell disease, multiple myeloma and in patients with leukopenia. Fever may also occur in pernicious anaemia and Hodgkin's disease.
2. The patient may have had a gastrectomy or a resection of the small bowel.
3. Jaundice may indicate haemolysis. In the inherited haemolytic anaemias jaundice may be present from birth. Jaundice may also result from liver cirrhosis and portal hypertension.
4. Diabetes may rarely be secondary to haemochromatosis or associated with pernicious anaemia.
5. Secondary polycythaemia may be associated with chronic lung disease.

EXAMINATION

Q7.7 What are the non-specific signs of anaemia?

A: • Pallor of mucous membranes.[1]
- Tachycardia.
- Full volume pulse.
- Systolic ejection murmur.
- Ankle oedema.
- Congestive cardiac failure.

1. Skin pallor is not a reliable sign of anaemia.

Q7.8 Which areas of the body should be carefully examined in patients with diseases of the blood?

A: • Skin.[1]
- Nails.[2]
- Skull.[3]

- Fundus oculi.[4]
- Mouth.[5]
- Abdomen including anus and rectum.[6]
- Lymphoreticular system.
- Cardiovascular system.[5]
- Central nervous system.[8]
- Joints.[9]

1. See Q7.9.
2. Nails may show evidence of pallor, koilonychia and brittleness. Koilonychia is found in iron deficiency anaemia.
3. Changes in skull configuration may be seen in thalassaemia, sickle-cell disease and other inherited haemolytic anaemias due to extramedullary haemopoiesis.
4. Retinal haemorrhages may be visible in patients with thrombocytopenia, severe anaemia and acute leukaemias.
5. See Q7.10.
6. Hepatomegaly and splenomegaly are found in a variety of blood disorders. The anus is prone to infection and ulceration in patients with leukopenia. A patient with iron deficiency anaemia may have haemorrhoids or a carcinoma of rectum.
7. Severe anaemia may be complicated by congestive cardiac failure.
8. Deficiency of vitamin B_{12} may be complicated by subacute combined degeneration of the cord. The central nervous system may be involved in acute leukaemia and lymphoma producing headache, signs of meningeal irritation and paraplegia.
9. Arthritic changes may result from bleeding into joints in haemophilia, gout may complicate chronic granulocytic leukaemia, and painful joint swelling may be seen in the Henoch–Schönlein syndrome.

Q7.9 What signs may be seen in the skin?

A: • Pallor.
- Purpura (petechial haemorrhages[1] and ecchymoses[2]).

- Telangiectasia.[3]
- Increased pigmentation.[4]
- Vitiligo.[5]
- Plethora of face.[6]
- Central cyanosis.[7]
- Jaundice.[8]
- Infection.
- Infiltration of skin by tumour cells.
- Ulceration.[9]
- Herpes zoster.[10]

1. Pinpoint haemorrhages into skin that do not blanch on pressure.
2. Larger confluent areas of blood within the skin (bruises).
3. Small dilated blood vessels that blanch on pressure. Look carefully for them on the lips.
4. Increased pigmentation may be associated with haemochromatosis or haemosiderosis.
5. Sometimes associated with pernicious anaemia.
6. Seen in polycythaemia in white-skinned patients.
7. May be associated with methaemoglobinaemia.
8. Seen in haemolytic and megaloblastic anaemias.
9. Sometimes seen in the legs of patients with sickle-cell disease and other haemolytic disorders such as hereditary spherocytosis.
10. Herpes zoster may be seen in chronic lymphocytic leukaemia.

Q7.10 What signs may be seen in the mouth?

A:
- Angular stomatitis (cheilosis).[1]
- Glossitis, atrophy of papillae.[2]
- Candidiasis.[3]
- Ulceration of mouth and fauces.[3]
- Herpes simplex.[3]
- Bleeding into gums.
- Gum hypertrophy.[4]

1. Cracking of the skin at the corner of the mouth may be due to iron or vitamin B_{12} deficiency. (It may, however, also be due to ill-fitting dentures!)

2. The tongue may be pale or red and painful in various forms of anaemia and deficiency diseases. In iron deficiency anaemia, glossitis, may be associated with dysphagia due to pharyngeal webs.
3. Conditions that may be seen in immunocompromised patients and in aplastic anaemia.
4. May be seen in acute leukaemias.

Q7.11 What features are common to all haemolytic anaemias irrespective of cause?

A: • Reticulocytosis.
• Erythroid hyperplasia of bone marrow.
• Increased serum bilirubin.
• Excess urinary urobilinogen.

LYMPHADENOPATHY

Q7.12 Lymphadenopathy may be found in a wide variety of disorders including many blood diseases. **Which sites should be examined in a systematic manner for evidence of lymphadenopathy?**

A: • Occipital.
• Submandibular.
• Cervical.
• Axillary.
• Epitrochlear.
• Inguinal.[1]
• Popliteal.

1. Small nodes may be of little clinical significance, being related to past infection in the extremities. This is especially true of nodes in the inguinal region.

Q7.13 If lymphadenopathy is present what should be noted?

A: • Site(s) affected.
• Number of nodes.
• Diameter of nodes.

- Consistency.
- Discrete or confluent.
- Mobile or fixed.
- Painful.
- Condition of overlying skin.

8
THE JOINTS

INTRODUCTION

SYMPTOMS

Q8.1 What are the major symptoms of joint disease?

A: • Pain.[1]
    • Swelling.
    • Stiffness.[2]
    • Limitation of movement.[3]

1. In most joint diseases pain has an aching quality but in gout it may be particularly severe and of a much sharper quality. Pain may also radiate widely. Pain arising from the hip, for example, is felt most often in the groin, but may radiate down the anterior aspect of the thigh to the knee, or be felt only in the knee; pain from the cervical spine may be felt in the shoulder, forearm and hand, and pain arising in the shoulder joint over the deltoid region.
2. Stiffness in rheumatoid arthritis and other inflammatory joint diseases is often most marked in the morning.
3. Loss of function should be assessed by inquiring about the patient's ability to carry out everyday tasks such as dressing. Patients may vary in their response to similar degrees of pain.

Q8.2 What features of joint pain should be noted?

A: • Duration.
    • Onset.[1]

- Characteristics.[2]
- Precipitating factors.[3]

1. Enquire whether onset of pain was sudden or gradual.
2. Enquire about severity, e.g. if it disturbs sleep, its radiation, and relationship to exercise and rest. Inflammatory joint pain (e.g. rheumatoid arthritis and ankylosing spondylitis) is worse after periods of inactivity in contrast to the pain of degenerative joint disease which is aggravated by exercise.
3. Injury, sore throat, diuretic therapy and other drugs, dietary indiscretion, sexual exposure and diarrhoea may precede the onset of pain.

FAMILY/SOCIAL/DRUG HISTORY

Q8.3 In the social history what points should be noted?

A: • Dietary history.[1]
  - Alcohol intake.[1]
  - Living conditions.[2]
  - Occupation.[3]
  - Sporting activities.[4]
  - Family history of joint disease, bleeding disorders or psoriasis.
  - Sexual activity.[5]

1. Dietary indiscretion and excessive alcohol intake may precede onset of acute gout.
2. Acute rheumatic fever is often associated with poor living conditions. Living upstairs may seriously affect mobility of arthritic patients.
3. Locomotor problems may result from occupational factors or may seriously affect patient's ability to work.
4. Osteoarthritis may follow sports injury.
5. Reiter's syndrome may follow sexually transmitted diseases. Gonorrhoea and HIV infection are also associated with arthritis.

Q8.4 What drugs may be associated with onset of arthralgia and arthritis?

A: • Penicillin and other antibiotics.[1]

- Hydralazine.[2]
- Procainamide.[2]
- Thiazide diuretics.[3]
- Drugs of addiction, e.g. heroin.[4]

1. May be followed by serum sickness.
2. May be associated with the development of systemic lupus erythematosus.
3. May precipitate gout.
4. Intravenous administration may lead to septic arthritis.

PAST MEDICAL HISTORY

Q8.5 What points should be noted in the past medical history?

A:
- Trauma.
- Recent sore throat.
- Recent bacterial diarrhoeal illness.[1]
- Tuberculosis and other infections.
- Sexually transmitted diseases.
- Psoriasis.
- Sickle-cell disease.
- Bleeding disorders.
- Ulcerative colitis or Crohn's disease.
- Diabetes.[2]

1. Certain shigella, salmonella, yersinia and campylobacter infections may be followed by a sterile inflammatory polyarthritis.
2. May be associated with frozen shoulder, stiffness of the fingers (cheiropathy) and rarely neuropathic joints.

EXAMINATION

Q8.6 What general features should be noted in patients with locomotor or joint disease before more detailed examination?

A:
- General appearance.[1]
- Posture and spine.[2]

- Limbs.[3]
- Gait.[4]
- Use of walking aid.
- Ability to sit and rise from a chair.
- Ability to undress, untie shoe laces, etc.

1. Rheumatoid arthritis and other joint diseases may be associated with constitutional symptoms. Does the patient look well or ill? Are there rashes? Look carefully for evidence of skin disease.
2. Look, for example, for evidence of scoliosis (lateral curvature of spine), angular kyphosis of the dorsal spine due to tuberculosis, increased kyphosis of the dorsal spine due to osteoporosis and the characteristic stoop of ankylosing spondylitis.
3. Are there, for example, valgus or varus deformities of the arms and legs (deviations away from and towards the mid-line of the limbs)?
4. Abnormal gaits may result from (i) joint disease, (ii) abnormalities of long bones due, for example, to shortening, (iii) neurological disease, (iv) muscle disease, or (v) wearing of prosthesis.

Q8.7 How should clinical examination of joints be carried out?

A: • Inspection.[1]
   • Palpation.
   • Testing range of movement in a systematic manner and by comparing joint mobility on both sides of the body.[2]

1. Start, for example, with hands then proceed to examine wrists, elbows, shoulders, temporomandibular joints, spine, hips and joints of lower limbs.
2. Passive testing of the range of joint movement may be more informative than active testing, but test gently. If possible, it is helpful to measure movement in degrees from a neutral or zero position, i.e. when the body is in the classic anatomical position. Test the following movements: flexion, extension, abduction, adduction,

rotation when applicable and, in the spine, lateral flexion.

Q8.8 What should be observed on inspection of joints?

A:
- Pattern of joint involvement.[1]
- Joint swelling and inflammation.
- Pattern of deformity.
- Muscle wasting around joint.
- Changes in overlying skin.

1. For example, which joints are affected and is involvement symmetrical?

Q8.9 What are the signs of acute inflammation of joints?

A:
- Redness of overlying skin.[1]
- Swelling.[2]
- Warmth.
- Tenderness.
- Limitation of movement.

1. Overlying skin may be moist in septic arthritis and rheumatic fever, and dry in gout.
2. Swelling may not be seen in inflammatory lesions of the shoulders, hips, sacroiliac joints and spine.

Q8.10 What points should be noted on palpation of joints?

A:
- Tenderness.[1]
- Nature of joint swelling.[2]
- Crepitus.[3]
- Presence of nodules, osteophytes, tophi.

1. Distinguish between tenderness arising from the joint and extra-articular structures.
2. See Q8.11.
3. May be a sign of osteoarthritis and can often be appreciated by passive flexion and extension of knee.

Q8.11 What may cause joint swelling?

A: • Fluid.[1]
   • Thickening of synovium.[2]
   • Bony enlargement.[3]

1. Fluid can be demonstrated by fluctuation or, in the knee joint, by tapping the patella.
2. Synovial thickening has a firm, non-fluctuant 'boggy' feel.
3. Bony enlargements (Heberden's nodes) may frequently be seen in distal interphalangeal joints, or at the proximal interphalangeal joints (Bouchard's nodes). Thickening of the ends of bones occurs in hypertrophic pulmonary osteoarthropathy.

Q8.12 What deformities may be seen in the hands and wrists of a patient with rheumatoid arthritis?

A: • Swelling of proximal interphalangeal joints.[1]
   • Swelling of metacarpophalangeal (MP) joints.
   • Subluxation of MP joints.
   • Thickening of the flexor tendons.
   • Ulnar deviation of fingers at MP joints.
   • 'Swan neck' deformity of fingers.[2]
   • 'Boutonnière' deformity of fingers.[3]
   • Muscle wasting.
   • Swelling of extensor and flexor synovium at the wrist.

1. Distal interphalangeal joints are involved in 30% of cases. Psoriatic arthropathy and gout, however, can affect any of the joints of the hand.
2. Hyperextension of proximal and flexion of distal interphalangeal (IP) joints.
3. Flexion of proximal and extension of distal IP joints.

Q8.13 What signs may be found in the hands of a patient with osteoarthritis?

A: • Involvement of the distal interphalangeal joints (Heberden's nodes).
   • Involvement of the proximal interphalangeal joints (Bouchard's nodes).

- Involvement of the carpometacarpal joint of the thumb.

Q8.14 What is a Baker's cyst?

A: A Baker's cyst may form in the popliteal fossa in patients with rheumatoid arthritis. It results from expansion of the synovial space. If the joint ruptures the synovial fluid may enter the calf producing a clinical picture resembling a deep venous thrombosis.

Q8.15 What skin lesions may be seen in patients with joint disease?

A:
- Pallor.[1]
- Vasculitic lesions.[2]
- Leg ulcers.[3]
- Livedo reticularis.[4]
- Sclerosis of skin.[5]
- Telangiectasia.[5]
- Raynaud's phenomenon.[6]
- Erythematous butterfly rash.[7]
- Photosensitivity.[7]
- Purpura.[7]
- Urticaria.[7]
- Alopecia.[7]
- Rash of dermatomyositis.
- Keratoderma blennorrhagica.[8]
- Erythema marginatum.[9]
- Erythema nodosum.[10]

1. Anaemia is common in rheumatoid arthritis.
2. Cutaneous infarctions due to vasculitis may be seen in systemic lupus erythematosus and rheumatoid arthritis.
3. A common problem in the legs of patients with rheumatoid arthritis.
4. Evidence of vasculitis in systemic lupus erythematosus and rheumatoid arthritis.
5. Seen in systemic sclerosis (scleroderma).
6. Seen in connective tissue diseases, particularly systemic sclerosis.

7. Seen in systemic lupus erythematosus.
8. Seen in post-venereal Reiter's syndrome.
9. One of the major criteria for the diagnosis of rheumatic fever.
10. Erythema nodosum may be associated with arthritis, although its more common associations are with a variety of infectious diseases, sarcoidosis and certain drugs.

Q8.16 What signs may be seen in the eyes?

A:
- Conjunctivitis.[1]
- Iritis.[2]
- Scleritis.[3]
- Scleromalacia.[4]
- Retinopathy.[5]

1. Conjunctivitis is one of the triad of features of Reiter's syndrome, the others being a seronegative reactive arthritis and non-specific urethritis. It is also common in rheumatoid arthritis as a result of a reduction in the secretion of tears. Sjögren's syndrome consists of rheumatoid arthritis, dry eyes (keratoconjunctivitis sicca) and a dry mouth (xerostomia). It may also be found in other diseases of connective tissue.
2. Seen in ankylosing spondylitis and juvenile chronic arthritis.
3. Scleritis causes a painful red eye, and is a poor prognostic sign.
4. In scleromalacia the sclera has a bluish tinge around the iris.
5. Retinopathy may be seen in systemic lupus erythematosus.

Q8.17 What signs of involvement of the cardiovascular system may be seen?

A:
- Pericarditis and pericardial effusion.[1]
- Hypertension.[2]
- Involvement of heart valves.[3]

1. Seen in systemic lupus erythematosus and rheumatoid arthritis.
2. Hypertension complicates many cases of polyarteritis nodosa and systemic sclerosis.
3. Valve lesions may occur in systemic lupus erythematosus. Aortic regurgitation has been described in association with ankylosing spondylitis.

Q8.18 What abnormalities may be found in the lungs?

A:
- Pleural effusion.[1]
- Fibrosing alveolitis.[2]
- Pulmonary nodules.[3]
- Aspiration pneumonia.[4]

1. Seen in patients with rheumatoid arthritis and systemic lupus erythematsus (SLE).
2. Lower lobe fibrosis is a feature of systemic sclerosis, and occurs in rheumatoid arthritis and systemic lupus erythematosus.
3. Nodule(s) may rarely occur in the lungs of patients with rheumatoid arthritis.
4. May complicate systemic sclerosis due to involvement of the oesophagus.

Q8.19 What neurological disorders may be seen?

A:
- Psychiatric disorders.[1]
- Epilepsy.[1]
- Cerebrovascular accident.[1]
- Cranial nerve lesions.[1]
- Peripheral neuropathy.[1]
- Cervical cord compression.[2]
- Carpal tunnel syndrome.[3]

1. Neurological complications that may be seen in systemic lupus erythematosus. Peripheral neuropathy may also complicate rheumatoid arthritis and polyarteritis nodosa.
2. A serious complication resulting from involvement of the atlantoaxial joint in rheumatoid arthritis. It may also occur in patients with cervical spondylosis.
3. Seen commonly in rheumatoid arthritis.